Truth About Nutrition

Dr. Joel D. Wallach, BS, DVM, ND

Copyright © 2016 Dr. Joel D. Wallach, BS, DVM, ND

All rights reserved.

Contents

CHAPTER 1 1
WHO IS DR. JOEL D. WALLACH, BS, DVM, ND?
The Modern Paradox 1
My Story 2
What Animals Taught Me 5
My Mission Today 10
Message Goes Global 13
Good Food/Bad Food 13
Good Foods 14
Bad Foods 17
Additional Bad Foods
(and More Information) for Diabetics 19
A Word About Phytates 20
Hyperthyroidism and Hypothyroidism 21

CHAPTER 2 23
A PRIMER ON MEDICINE
Immortal You 23
Regulating Life Span 24
Doctors Are Not Wizards 26
Various Medical Specialties 28
A Word About "Orthodox" Physicians................................29
We Can Do Better Than That! 31
The ABCs of Diseases and Their Cures 32
What Are Essential Nutrients? 48
So What's the Argument? 50

CHAPTER 3 53
WHY DO WE NEED SUPPLEMENTS?

What to Expect 53
What Are Minerals? 54
We Are Not Carrots 55
Soil Depletion 56

CHAPTER 4 59
WHAT DOES LONGEVITY LOOK LIKE?

Do You Want to Live to Be 100?.....................................59
An Animal Model for Longevity......................................60
The Human Model for Longevity....................................61
Fourteen Hunza Secrets..64
What We Know About the Human Model.......................66
What Are Centenarians?...67
Meet the Centenarians!..68
Centenarians Are Amazing!..68
Eight Model Cultures...73
The Common Good..74
The Scorecard..75

CHAPTER 5 79
MISPLACED TRUST

The Healthcare Buck..79
It's No Laughing Matter..82
The End of Managed Healthcare.....................................83
Lying to Insurance Companies..85
Carpenter With No Hammer Skills..................................88
Dead or Alive..89
Who Do You Trust?..90
Talk About a Revolution...92

CHAPTER 6 97
MISINFORMATION ABOUNDS
The Yolk's on Us..97
Could Alzheimer's Disease Be Doctor Inflicted? 101
This Raises My Blood Pressure...103
What Price Menopause?...107
But Weight…There's More!..109

CHAPTER 7 113
THREE SERIOUS TOPICS
Cancer, War, and Lies..113
The Diabetes Epidemic: Who's to Blame?.........................120
Make No Bones About It..123
Pour the Soda Pop Down the Drain...................................128
In Conclusion..129

DISCLAIMER

Note that this book is not intended as a substitute for the medical advice of physicians. The publisher of this book and its associates do not dispense medical advice or prescribe the use of any technique as a form of treatment for medical problems, either directly or indirectly, without the advice of a physician. In the event that you use any of the information in this book for yourself, which is your constitutional right, the publisher of this book and its associates assume no responsibility for your actions.

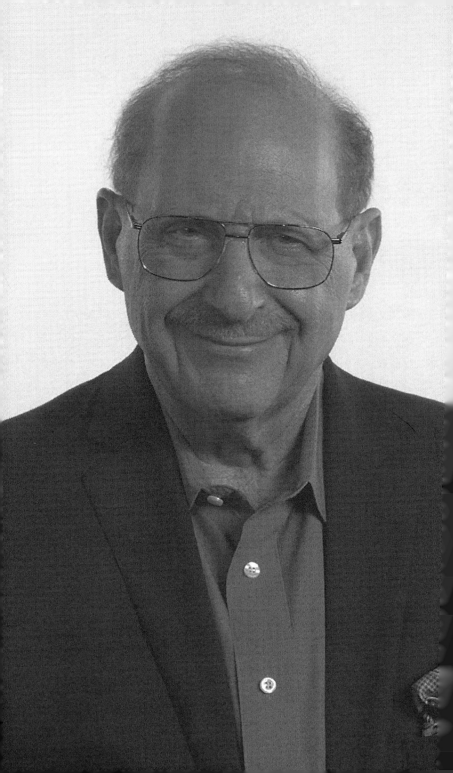

CHAPTER 1

Who Is Dr. Joel D. Wallach, BS, DVM, ND?

The Modern Paradox

Every year, we seem to progress in leaps and bounds in medical breakthroughs and scientific discovery. However, the occurrence of degenerative diseases continues to climb at an alarming rate! Every year, researchers produce more and more studies and continue to give additional advice about how to live longer and healthier. Yet, every year, as a whole, we are far less healthy. This is one of the great paradoxes of modern living.

The truth about nutrition isn't something recently produced in a lab nor something yet to be discovered. The truth has been right under our noses. Even as a young farm boy, the truth showed itself to me in plain sight!

Researchers have figured out how to use stem cells to create artificial organs. But we can't seem to stop the increase in the number one killer: cardiovascular disease.

One in three Americans has diabetes. This is largely due to the dramatic increase in obesity.

This declining health comes at a time when environmental and day-to-day stress has risen dramatically. More than ever, we need maximum health and vitality. As a whole, we are nutritionally deficient and over-drugged and on the wrong track, and most of us are without a clue as to how or why.

THIS IS WHERE I COME IN.

My Story

Now, if any of you grew up on a farm or have anything to do with livestock, then you are my kind of people. I grew up on a beef farm in West St. Louis County in Missouri. And if you raise livestock, for those of you without that experience, your chance of making money is better if you raise your own feed. So, we raised our own corn and our own soybeans and our own hay.

We had a truck come down from the mill, and this truck would grind up the corn, soybeans and hay, and then we would add sacks of vitamins and minerals, and we'd make pellets out of it, and this is what we would feed the calves. Then, in six months' time, we'd ship them to market to be slaughtered, and we'd save back some of the best ones for ourselves, and we'd knock them on the head and eat them, to put it bluntly.

It always fascinated me, as a teenager, that we did that for those calves, and then in six months, we'd ship them off to be slaughtered or we'd eat them. Yet, we wanted to live to be a hundred years of age without any aches and pains, and guess what? We didn't take any vitamins or minerals, and that bothered me. So I asked my dad. I'd say, "Hey, Pops. How come we do that for those calves, but we don't do that for us?" And he'd give me that good old-fashioned Missouri farm wisdom. He'd say things like, "Shut up, boy. You're getting this farm-fresh food, and free exercise. Don't ask complicated questions." And, of course, I was very quiet then because I didn't want to miss out on any meals.

Well, when I went to school, I went to the University of Missouri, the School of Agriculture, and I got my degree in Agriculture. My major was in Animal Husbandry and Nutrition. My minor was in Field Crops and Soils. My Soils professor and mentor, Dr. William Albrecht, was a legend in agronomy and the foremost authority on the relation of soil fertility to human health. He taught that there was a direct link to infertile soils and degenerative diseases in animals and in humans. The soils in farms were becoming depleted of many of the essential minerals that animals and humans require for good health. However, the farmers were only fertilizing the soils with the very short list of minerals attributed to higher yields. The overall nutrition of the crops was declining in value. This is a problem that still exists to this day.

Mineral deficient soils producing mineral deficient plants is the reason farmers need to give mineral supplements to their livestock, just as I did with my dad as a boy.

The pieces began coming together. I was receiving intensive training on matters of soils and minerals and their direct relationship with the healthfulness of livestock. My pathology mentor, Loren Kintner, taught me to be extremely thorough in my pathology work and to continue to ask questions. And after entering veterinary school, I soon learned the answer to my age-old question to my dad as to why the farmers supplemented their livestock and there wasn't much interest in supplementing themselves and their families.

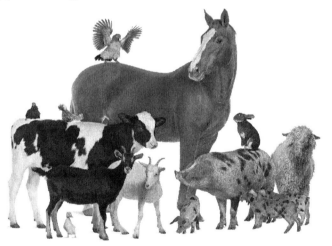

The answer is this. We know how to prevent and cure diseases in animals with nutrition, and the reason why we do that is because farmers don't have major-medical, we don't have hospitalization, we don't have Blue Cross and Blue Shield, we don't have Medicare, we don't have Obama to watch out for us. If you're going to make money as a farmer, you'd better know how to do stuff yourself. You'd better care for your animals efficiently and effectively with feed and nutrition, if you can.

To some, the possibility that human nutrition would ever be given such attention seemed impossible. But my life on the farm had taught me to believe that impossible just takes a little bit longer.

Well, to make a long story short, after I got out of veterinary school, I went to Africa for two years and was able to fulfill a boyhood dream. I became a Frank Buck for the two years and worked with Marlin Perkins. Many of you will remember him from the Mutual of Omaha's Wild Kingdom as a great gentleman.

After two years of working with elephants and rhinos, people used to ask me, "Are you a small-animal vet or a large-animal vet?" Well, I was telling them that I was an extra-large animal vet because I worked with elephants and rhinos. After some time, Marlin sent me a telegram and said, "Would you come back to the St. Louis Zoo and work with us? We need a wildlife veterinarian at the zoo for a special project. We were given a seven and a half million-dollar grant from the National Institutes of Health, and what we need is a veterinarian who will do autopsies of animals that die of natural causes in the zoo."

What Animals Taught Me

I was just overjoyed to do that. So I came back, and of course, I not only did autopsies for animals that died in the St. Louis Zoo, but the Brookfield Zoo in Chicago, the Bronx Zoo in New York, the National Zoo, the L.A. Zoo, and so forth. My job, again, was to do autopsies on animals that died of natural causes in the zoo and look for a species of animals that was ultra sensitive to pollution.

This was because, in the early sixties, we had just learned about pollution and ecological problems and disasters, and nobody knew quite what to do. So I was supposed to find a species of animals that was extra sensitive to this and use them much like we did the canaries in the mine. The old Welsh coal miners used to put a canary in a little wicker cage and take it down in the mine. And if methane gas or carbon monoxide would leak in the mine, the canary would drop off the perch and die first, and the men knew to get out before the mine blew up or they suffocated.

Again, to make a long story short, over a period of some twelve years, I did 17,500 autopsies in over 454 species of animals, and 3,000 human beings who lived in close proximity to zoos, and the thing that I found out was this: Every animal, and every human being, who dies of natural causes dies of a nutritional deficiency. Did you catch that? Those who die of a natural cause actually die of a nutritional deficiency. That fascinated me. Gee, isn't that fascinating? Everybody's dying of nutritional deficiencies, and we can document this at autopsy both chemically and biochemically, and so forth, with things that you study and see on the autopsy table.

You would think that, with such incredible discoveries, and especially since veterinarians have been successfully using nutritional supplements for decades to eliminate birth defects and increase the healthfulness and longevity of farm and zoo animals, there would be a surge of interest in using supplements to eliminate birth defects and reduce degenerative diseases across the human race! Remember, farmers used cost-effective strategies out of necessity, while insurance encouraged people to use more expensive (and less effective) strategies to maintain their own health. And the other side of that coin is that doctors could make more money by suggesting and using more expensive methods. In fact, doctors could essentially make more money using less effective methods. This is the crooked nature of the system. A doctor might make a few hundred dollars using nutrition to fix or prevent a degenerative disease, but they can make tens of thousands of dollars to continue to "manage" the disease. Not to mention the fact that the extra income doctors are accustomed to with added unnecessary surgeries, tests, and biopsies, and managing more and more side effects and other diseases as a result of not fixing the problems and, instead, managing diseases.

Progress all too often follows where the money is. Doctors would much rather use patients as ATM machines than to be broke while studying and promoting nutrition.

Doctors get paid when you are unwell, and they are out of a job when you are healthy. Despite these facts, many people such as my mentors and me were actively pursuing human and animal remedies with nutrition. However, the doctors were armed with lots of money and propaganda. They also leveraged the one great thing the medical community produced: antibiotics. Antibiotics were able to fix infectious diseases quickly. The results could not be refuted. Doctors made a lot of headway using antibiotics with the sick population. People began to attribute the success of antibiotics to the doctors' methods.

And they began to blindly follow every other bit of advice the doctors suggested.

Now, the doctors could promote drugs besides antibiotics, and patients would take them without so much as a smidgeon of hesitation. The money came pouring in, and it continues to do so. Doctors and pharmaceuticals are filling their pockets to the hilt while the masses' health declines and while patients experience side effects and lasting aches and pains, because the root problems to their diseases are not getting fixed.

While the basic studies of nutrition have become the neglected stepchild of the last century's science, the unquestionable basic mineral needs of our human flesh and bone cry out for attention from the waiting rooms of physicians' offices, hospital wards, operating tables, and morgues.

I did my part, but it was like banging my head against a brick wall. I wrote 75 scientific articles. I wrote eight multi-authored textbooks, and one textbook of my own that cost one hundred and forty bucks for medical students, and I'm sure the only thing they use them for are doorstops. I couldn't get anyone excited. I was in 1,700 newspapers, I was in magazines, I was on "20/20" and every other network TV show that you can think of, and guess what? I couldn't get anyone excited back in the 1960s about nutrition.

So the veterinarian was on his way to becoming a naturopathic physician.

HAVE YOU HEARD OF A NATUROPATHIC PHYSICIAN?

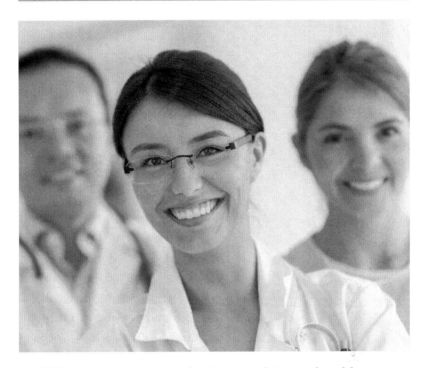

An ND is a primary care physician and is regulated by a state medical board much like MDs are. Naturopathic physicians can do virtually everything that an MD can, and in addition, they can do other things such as acupuncture, prescribe herbs, and offer nutritional counseling. Yet many in the orthodox medical profession looked upon naturopathy as a strange, old-fashioned offshoot of medicine bordering on quackery. Naturopathic physicians, in turn, looked upon the traditional medical community as uncaring, arrogant, heavy-handed upstarts who over-prescribe drugs with harmful side effects, perform unnecessary surgery out of greed, and deliver unnecessary chemotherapy and radiation out of ignorance.

I had come to a professional juncture here. Do I totally give up on twenty years of orthodox research and association with the mainstream of science and join this maverick band of healthcare professionals? Members of the medical community were rolling in money. But they weren't fixing problems, and they'd set aside research on nutrition. I realized it would be an uphill battle trying to bring my veterinarian expertise into the mainstream path of the MDs. A door opened for me to become a naturopath, and I was ready for my next adventure. I knew that physicians could see patients. And that was enough, because I knew that the philosophy I learned about preventing diseases in animals would work on humans, too!

My Mission Today

My mission today is to apply all that I have learned about nutrition and animal studies to humans. I want to help all of us live longer and in better health.

I want to meet the paradox of modern living head on.

We have the knowledge, and we have the right nutritional products. We have the successful trials and documented research. We have hundreds of thousands of people who have already stood up to their doctors saying they have had enough. It is up to each of us to study the research, and to apply the nutritional techniques and enjoy a healthier and longer life. If we can stop listening to our medical doctors, who have their own agendas, we can live longer and healthier. If we give our bodies the raw materials they need, we can heal ourselves. The body can fix itself naturally when it gets everything that it needs.

THIS IS MY CRUSADE.

My crusade is to get the word out on how to prevent and reverse degenerative diseases. Many humans all over the world are at the end of their ropes. Doctors say there's nothing more that can be done for them, except maybe some more pain management and more tests and more radiation.

We just apply the simple facts that we've learned in the animal industry to our human patients, and it never fails. It always works. It's up to each of us to make the choice.

OUR FUTURE IS IN OUR HANDS.

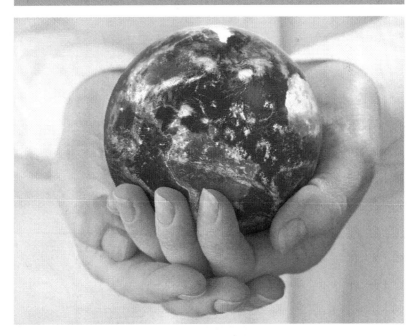

Ultimately, we are what's in (or isn't in) the food we eat and what we absorb. Therefore, it matters not whether one follows the concepts of the Beverly Hills Diet, the South Beach Atkins Diet, the Fit for Life Diet, the Mediterranean Diet, Dr. Berger's Immune Power Diet, Pritikin Diet, the Macrobiotic Diet, Pearson's and Shaw's Life Extension Diet, or the 120 Year Diet or the See Food Diet (when you see food, you eat it).

It doesn't matter if you become a vegan or remain a carnivore.

It doesn't matter whether you eat blubber like an Eskimo or eat dozens of burgers each day like Wimpy, the original "junk food junkie" from Popeye cartoons.

It doesn't matter whether you eat a pound of tofu or bean sprouts or avocados each day, either. It doesn't matter if you raise your own herbs in your backyard greenhouse and only eat organic veggies and grass-fed beef. It doesn't matter if you are one of the world's most avid juicers.

If you don't supplement your diet daily with optimal amounts of each of the 90 essential nutrients (according to your body weight), you're throwing away 50% to 75% of your life as surely as if you've jumped in front of a speeding commuter train—purposely.

And you'll get the same results as if you'd stepped in front of that train.

Hopefully, you will make the right choice.

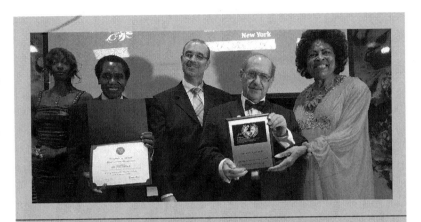

Message Goes Global

In August of 2015, Dr. Wallach was selected to receive the prestigious Global Official of Dignity Award at the WCH Humanitarian Summit in New York City. He was presented the international award at the United Nations headquarters in the presence of royalties, dignitaries, and luminaries from business, academe, government, and entertainment fields who are honorees and delegations from around the world. That's right. Dr. Wallach's message about nutrition and health has reached around the world.

Good Food/Bad Food

It's important to supplement your diet with the 90 essential nutrients every day. But if you eat the wrong foods while you supplement your diet, and you don't eat the right foods, then you still won't maximize your potential for longevity.

In other words, to get the full benefits from the 90 essential nutrients, you must eat the right foods, and you must avoid the wrong foods. Some foods will decrease your ability to absorb the 90 essential nutrients. And, when you eat those foods, you are hindering the good that you are trying to do.

There's no workaround. Supplement right and eat right, and you'll live longer and healthier. Eat wrong and don't supplement, and you will not.

If you are serious about your health, this lifestyle change is a must. You will then ensure you are getting the most out of your daily vitamin and mineral supplement regimen. It is easier than you think and the end result is very rewarding!

The Good Foods

Here are the good foods that will support your body's efforts to heal itself:

- **Eggs** – Should be a staple of your diet. They are considered by many as a super food. Not only do they contain vital cholesterol that your brain, nerves, and hormones need to function but they also contain a whole slew of proteins, EFA's, vitamins and minerals that help your body function. I recommend eating at least 6 eggs a day (for Alzheimer's and other dementias, I recommend you eat 10+ eggs a day to feed your brain the cholesterol it needs to function). Do not overcook eggs. Soft scramble them in butter and salt, soft boil them, poach them, or eat them raw in a smoothie. Note that there is a chance to get salmonella from the outside shell of the egg that was exposed to the cloaca of the chicken. If you are going to eat raw eggs, put a teaspoon of bleach into a quart of water and put the eggs into the solution, then dry them off, and they are ready to use. The bleach will kill off any microorganisms on the outside of the shell. If you hard-boil an egg and the yolk has a greenish coating, this means that the cholesterol has been degraded, so it is best to soft boil eggs. If you are allergic to chicken eggs, then you can try goose, duck, or quail eggs.

- **Butter** – Real butter, not the stuff that you can't believe isn't butter – because that stuff is not butter.

- **Iodized Salt** – Your body needs salt to create stomach acid. If you are on a salt restricted diet, you will not be able to create stomach acid causing acid reflux/heartburn. So use as much salt as you want, and salt your food to taste.

- **Dairy** – Full-fat whole milk only. No skim, 1 percent, or 2 percent milk.

- **Beef** – Rare or medium-rare only. Make sure there are no grill or char marks on your meat. Use a pressure cooker or crockpot.

- **Vegetables** – Do not stir fry your vegetables (see fried foods). Organically grown produce is not nutritionally better than conventionally grown. If you look at the requirements for produce to be labeled by the USDA as organic, you will be surprised to find that the produce must be grown from soil that has not had prohibited substances applied to it for only 3 years. So a field could have been sprayed with prohibited substances for 50 years, but if they stop spraying it with prohibited substances for 3 years, then it can be certified organic. Back in 1936, it was brought to our government's attention that our soils where horribly depleted through U.S. Senate Document #264. So no matter what you eat, organic or conventional, it is impossible to get all the nutrients your body needs every day from the food you eat.

- **Nuts** – Salted or mixed nuts are okay. Because most peanuts are contaminated with fungus, it is recommended you don't eat them. Do not eat nuts that have been processed on the same machines as wheat.

- **Nut Butters** – Are fine to eat as long as they have no extra sugar or oils. You can make your own oil- and sugar-free nut butters with a powerful blender.

- **Pure Buckwheat** – It isn't wheat.

- **Couscous** – Made from pearl millet only.

- **Corn** – Is one of the foods I suggest buying organic because most conventional corn is genetically modified which can hurt your digestive tract.

- **Unfiltered Water** – Four to eight 8 oz. glasses of water daily. Avoid soft plastic bottles and BPA. Avoid drinking tap water since most cities fluoridate their water. Fluoride has been proven to reduce your IQ, motivation, and creativity. Recently, even Harvard University has released a study linking fluoride to "significantly lower" IQ scores. Do not drink any alkaline waters just before or while eating since it neutralizes your stomach acid like carbonated drinks which prevents digestion and absorption of nutrients.

- **Lard** – Use the real stuff from the butcher or rendered lard made at home. Avoid the lard products that have added oils and hydrogenated by-products.

- **Fish**

- **Chicken**

- **Pork**

- **Lamb**

- **Fruit**

- **Cooked Rice**

- **Millet**

- **Beans**

- **Quinoa**

- **Coffee**

- **Tea and Green Tea**

- **Red Wine**

The Bad Foods

Here are the bad foods that we all need to avoid no matter how many dietary supplements we might take:

- **Wheat**

- **Barley**

- **Rye**

- **Oats/Oatmeal** – The grains we eat today have been altered to withstand weather, insects, and weed killers. This has resulted in a gluten protein that our stomachs just cannot break down. When the gluten travels through our intestinal track undigested, it destroys the villi and micro-villi that is meant to absorb the nutrients from our foods. This leads to digestive, chronic health problems and diseases. The category of oats/oatmeal includes some alcoholic beverages. Avoid these grains even if it states on the package that they are gluten free.

- **Fried Food** – When you fry foods or overheat them, that produces acrylamides and free radicals. These carcinogens can lead to inflammation in your digestive track and arteries, and oxidation damage to your nerves and soft tissues, and they can cause certain cancers. This includes stir fried foods.

- **Oils** – Cooking oils, olive oil, and even coconut oil oxidizes when oxygen comes in contact with it. When you eat oxidized oil, it causes inflammation and oxidation damage, and it destroys tissues in your body. This category includes mayonnaise, salad dressings, fish packed in oils, and any food in oil. In nature, there is no cooking oil tree, and no spigot at the base of an olive tree to get oil from. So our bodies were just not designed to eat mass quantities of oils as we do today.

- **Well-Done Meat (Rare or Medium Rare is okay)** – Carcinogenic heterocyclic amines are created by high temperature cooking of meat. Make sure, when you're barbecuing, that you do not let the flames touch the meat, or let the juices from the meat hit the charcoal and coat the meat with smoke. Heterocyclic amines are the most egregious cancer causing substances on earth.

- **Deli Meats/Cold Cuts** – Most deli meats, hot dogs, and bacon have nitrates and nitrites in them as preservatives. Nitrites and nitrates cause inflammation, tissue destruction, oxidation, and free radical damage. If you can get nitrate/nitrite free deli meats, then they are okay to consume.

- **Carbonated Beverages** – Neutralize your stomach acid and reduce your ability to digest and absorb the nutrients from your food and supplements. Phosphoric acid is especially bad for you, and will rob calcium from your bones.

- **Potato/Yam/Sweet Potato Skins** – The skin is okay to eat only after you boil it.

Additional Bad Foods
(and More Information) for Diabetics

Besides eliminating the Bad Foods we all have to avoid, those of us with type 2 diabetes must also eliminate additional foods from our diet until we get our blood sugar levels normalized for four consecutive weeks without the help of prescription drugs. Some additional foods for diabetics to avoid:

- **Fruit**

- **Fruit Juice**

- **Dried Fruit**

- **Honey**

- **Agave Syrup**

- **Maple Syrup**

- **Stuff high in sugar or carbohydrates**

- **Molasses**

- **Alcohol**

- **Gluten Free Grains**

- **Grains**

When you have diabetes and you are eating whole grain bread instead of white bread, it's like you are shooting yourself with a copper-jacket bullet instead of a hollow point steel jacket.

A Word About Phytates

Foods with phytic acid include beans, seeds, and some nuts, but phytates* can turn up in other foods, too. It will bind to minerals in your foods or supplements and cause them not to be absorbed by your body. To avoid this, make sure you take your minerals two to three hours before or after you consume a meal with phytates. You can also cook foods with phytates to eliminate the harmful effects. Some examples of foods that contain phytates are: linseeds, sesame seeds, almonds, brazil nuts, coconuts, hazelnuts, peanuts, walnuts, corn, bran from rice (brown rice), pinto beans, chickpeas, hummus, lentils, soybeans, tofu, and spinach.

Hyperthyroidism and Hypothyroidism

Those with thyroid issues should avoid cruciferous vegetables altogether. Some common examples of cruciferous vegetables are: horseradish, kale, collard greens, cabbage, brussel sprouts, broccoli, cauliflower, bok choy, turnip, mustard seed, arugula, watercress, radish, and wasabi.

Foods with phytates are ok when cooked

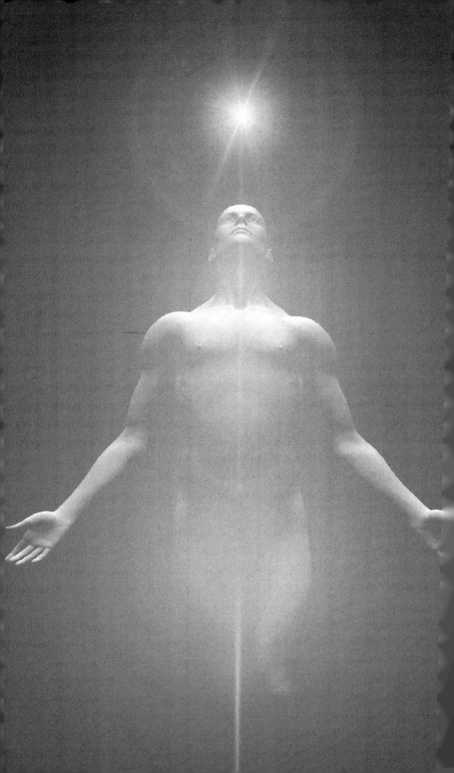

A PRIMER ON MEDICINE

Immortal You

Forget about making the choice to shorten your life span by relying on the nutrients in your diet and relying on the advice of your doctor instead of the research results. And let's forget, too, about eating the wrong foods instead of the good foods.

Let's talk about a happier possibility.

Have you ever wanted to be immortal? In a sense, we all are.

The human species is immortal.
Individuals age and die. But some of the cells in our bodies are part of a stream of cells that have been reproducing themselves since time began. These cells don't know what death is. They only know life, and for those cells, there is immortality.

Regulating Life Span

How can we live longer? There are three ways to increase maximum life span in laboratory animals. These laboratory animals are fed perfect diets with the perfect blend of vitamins and minerals.

1. Lower metabolic rate by a calorie restricted intake (without malnutrition)
2. Enhance antioxidant protection
3. Supplement with perfect blend of vitamins and minerals

The fact that we can increase life spans means that we do not have to age, sicken, and die on a particular schedule. We'll do that, however, if we depend on the foods we eat to give us all the nutrition we need to live long, healthy lives.

Most of us mistakenly depend on the random distribution of essential minerals in our food. Even with the best medical care, that isn't enough to keep us healthy and living longer. For human beings to reach our potential for longevity and health, we must become independent of our soil with its mineral and vitamin deficiencies. We need:

a. Supplements so that we have more predictable nutrition
b. Calorie restricted diets
c. A load of antioxidants

We also need constant oxygen, water, and essential macro and micro nutrients. We send people to the moon, but we still leave the essential nutritional intake of our cells and the building blocks of our enzymatic and physiological life on

Earth to blind chance.

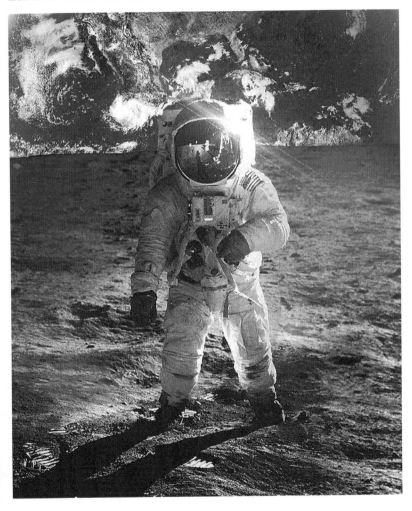

Does that make any sense at all?

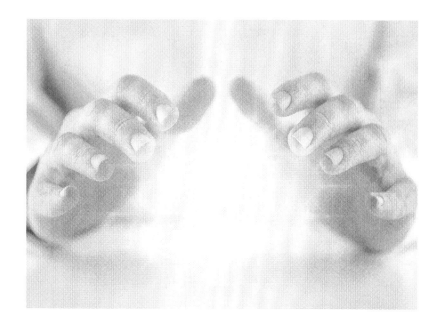

Doctors Are Not Wizards

What's wrong with doctors? For one thing, it's the healthcare system in this country. We do not have a free medical market in the United States. We have an uncontrolled and unrestrained medical monopoly that has led to these realities:

- Autism has risen from 1 out of 10,000 births to 1 out of 80. And yet autism is nothing more than a nutritional deficiency of the brain. It has nothing to do with genetics or vaccinations, just as ADD isn't a Ritalin deficiency.
- Alzheimer's has risen from obscurity to become the sixth leading cause of death.

- Heart disease, cancer, arthritis, high blood pressure, and obesity are out of control.

EVERYONE IS BECOMING SICKER ALL THE TIME.

Your medical doctor may be the nicest person in the world, but your medical doctor doesn't always know what's best for you. Doctors only know what they've been trained in. And what they've been trained in is one piece of the pie of medical science.

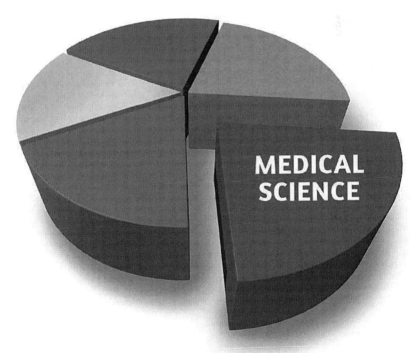

But the pharmaceutical industry—the health insurance, the monopoly, which is modern American medicine—has convinced everyone in the United States that medical doctors are the undisputed wizards of medicine, and they hold the answers to all the secrets of science.

It's just not true. I've reversed health problems in animals and in humans, and I can do it for you, too.

Various Medical Specialties

The type of medicine that your MD is trained in is called allopathic medicine. Your doctor is not trained in all medicine. Your doctor is trained in allopathic medicine.

Other practitioners may be trained in:

- Naturopathic medicine
- Chiropractic medicine
- Osteopathic medicine
- Homeopathic medicine

Each specialization is good for treating certain things. I go into detail about that in my book, Epigenetics.

Allopathic medicine, which is what your MD is trained in, is perfect for surgery, trauma care, and a handful of infectious diseases. That's the domain of the MD.

For all other conditions that people go to the doctor for—asthma, arthritis, high blood pressure, fibromyalgia, insomnia, depression, heartburn—allopathic medicine is the wrong key. It doesn't fit the lock. It doesn't work, and this is the single biggest secret there is in the United States or anywhere else in the world.

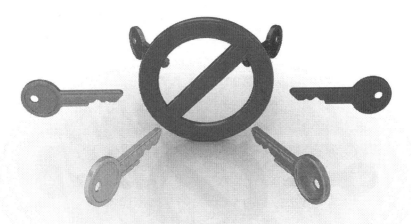

MD directed treatments for chronic diseases do not work. It is the wrong skill set for the job. The right skill set? Holistic, naturopathic therapeutics based on medical nutrition.

A Word About "Orthodox" Physicians

When I say "orthodox" physicians, I am not talking about the religious beliefs of doctors. I am referring to the fact that, as well-meaning as doctors might be, they are not impartial sources of information.

The information they would need to prevent, or cure, disease may be obvious. But, if that information would put them out of work or decrease their profits, they conveniently refuse to see the writing on the wall.

YOUR DOCTOR HAS AN AX TO GRIND.

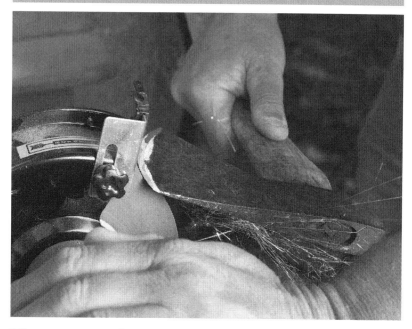

That means traditional physicians fail to know what any impartial researcher would have concluded through testing and through experience.

Orthodox physicians don't cure diseases because they want to hold onto their homes and their new Mercedes and their country club memberships. And they've enlisted your help in enriching their coffers! When you have the surgery, or submit yourself to the test, or take the prescription to the pharmacy, you're putting yourself in the hands of professionals who often put their interests, and their profits, before your health.

They use people as ATM machines. And they are financially motivated to manage the symptoms of a disease that never

goes away rather than getting rid of the disease. They make money when you are sick and not when you are well.
Does that philosophically sound as if it's in your best interest? The truth has been buried by popular yet incorrect theories that have made doctors and pharmaceutical companies rich.

We Can Do Better Than That!

Even if orthodox doctors don't want to find the answers, and they're not interested in the cures, that doesn't mean you have to believe there is no hope. Just look elsewhere for answers. You'll find more than 400 diseases and the alternative approach to treating them in my book, Dead Doctors Don't Lie. Along with all of the other suggestions, I assume you are consuming adequate amounts of the 90 essential nutrients daily. That is the starting point for good health for everyone.

Your president, governor, mayor, physician, or even your spouse can't do it for you.

You have to treat your body to the 90 essential nutrients that it needs. They will not be supplied in your diet alone.

Here are some examples of diseases and cures taken directly from my bestselling book, Dead Doctors Don't Lie, that you, or someone you love, might have now or in the future. This is just the abbreviated version of the first three letters of the alphabet in the alphabetized appendix of diseases taken from Dead Doctors Don't Lie.

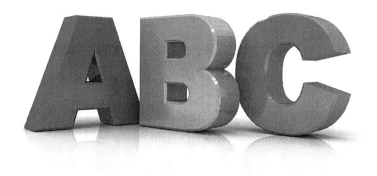

The ABCs of Diseases and Their Cures

ACNE (acne rosacea/acne vulgaris) is a frequent skin disease in teenagers and is sometimes associated with PMS and estrogen supplements during menopause. Papules, pustules, superficial pus-filled cysts, and deep pus-filled canals characterize acne. Acne is primarily the result of an essential fatty acid deficiency with a concurrent intake of too much saturated fat and polyunsaturated fatty acids (fried foods and margarine). Eliminate fast foods and other sources of fat and sugar. Check out the possibility of food allergies (i.e., wheat, milk, and soy) as a contributing factor. Betaine HCl and pancreatic enzymes are of considerable benefit. Essential fatty acids are a must and should be consumed at the rate of 3% of your total daily calorie consumption or supplemented at the rate of 9 grams per day in capsule form. A regimen of Vitamin A 300,000 units/day (as beta-carotene) for five months, then reduce to 25,000 units/day, B6 100 mg tid, zinc 50 mg tid for 30 days, and vitamin E oil applied topically to acne lesions is also recommended. Exposing areas affected by acne directly to ultraviolet light directly for 1 to 6 minutes may also prove helpful.

AGE SPOTS Also called liver spots or pigments of aging, these unsightly and embarrassing brown spots are caused by rancid fat from cell walls accumulating under your skin. If you have just ten age spots on the back of your hand, think how many millions you have in your vital organs: your brain, heart, liver, kidney, and lungs!

They interfere with cell function, shorten your life, and are a warning of a high risk of cancer and heart disease.

The good news is that age spots are reversible. When they go away on the outside, they go away on the inside, too.

Treatment includes eliminating all fried foods, vegetable oils, and sugar from your diet. Take selenium at 500 mcg per day, vitamin E at 1,200 IU, and all the other 90 essential nutrients.

ALOPECIA (baldness). Loss of hair, which can occur either partially or completely, can result from male-pattern baldness, female-pattern baldness, or alopecia universalis.

If you catch it early enough, under certain circumstances, you might find commercially available Minoxidil and Retin-A creams helpful in treating the condition and maintaining your regrown hair.

Deficiencies of the mineral tin have been shown to cause male-pattern baldness in laboratory animals. In fact, a plant-derived liquid colloidal tin helped me regrow my own hair.

ALOPECIA that occurs with eczema is often caused by essential fatty acid deficiency and can be treated with IV interlipids and/or oral flaxseed oil at the rate of 9 grams per day. Zinc at 50 mg tid is also indicated. Eliminating wheat and cow's milk from the diet will increase the rate of recovery. Ingesting HCI and pancreatic enzymes at 75 - 200 mg tid 15 - 20 minutes before meals are also important.

ANGINA This is a sharp, debilitating pain in the front and center of the chest from arterial disease in the heart which reduces the heart's oxygen supply. Symptoms may appear after strenuous exercise, simply climbing stairs, or after a meal.

The allopathic approach is the coronary bypass surgery which, after 20 years of study, has failed to be proven to prevent second heart attacks or to extend life. All that coronary bypass surgeries have been proven to do is to enrich the coffers of the cardiovascular surgeon!

So here's a better plan. Chelation, either IV with H202 and calcium EDTA or orally with vitamin/mineral and herb supplements, or the Dean Ornish diet can effect a cure over time. Avoid sugar, caffeine, and cigarette smoke. Exercise in the form of walking 30 minutes each day is very helpful. Calcium (2000 mg/day) and magnesium (800 mg/day) and essential fatty acids can help prevent progress of current disease, and reduce vitamin D intake from the sun and supplements. Nitroglycerin sublingual capsules and time-release transdermal patches are very useful in relieving symptoms. English hawthorn (Crataegus oxyacantha) and ginko (Ginko bilboa) are specific for relieving angina by increasing blood flow through coronary arteries.

The bottom line: Lifestyle changes and proper supplementation can reverse cardiovascular disease!

ANOREXIA (loss of appetite). Can be caused by stress, malnutrition, shock, and injury. "Orthodox" doctors like to think of anorexia as a psychiatric disease. However, it now appears that it is a manifestation of a severe food allergy.

A common complaint of anorexics is "I always feel better when I don't eat, and I feel bad when I do eat." Deficiencies of zinc and lithium are associated with anorexia. Elimination diets and pulse tests are useful in finding the offending food which is frequently cow's milk, wheat, eggs, and corn.

Treatment should include betaine HCl and pancreatic enzymes at a rate of 150 - 250 mg/day tid, and also the baseline vitamin and mineral supplements. Herbs are excellent appetite stimulants. Test herbal preparations of buckbean or marsh trefoil (Menyanthes trifoliata), centaury (Centaurium umbellatum), sweet flag or calamus (Acorus calamus), or yellow gentian (Gentiana lutea). All of the herbal preparations should be taken before meals. In the case of anorexia nervosa, autoimmune urine therapy may be indicated.

ANOSMIA (loss of smell). This can temporarily be caused

by colds or rhinitis (nasal inflammation from colds or allergy). Chronic loss of smell is most frequently the result of a zinc deficiency. However, in the cases of injury, stroke, or tumor, zinc supplements may not be effective.

ANXIETY (panic attacks). These affect women twice as frequently as men. This isn't surprising when you consider the total hormone biorhythm charts of women.

The base cause can be either a food allergy reaction (i.e., corn, cow's milk, wheat, etc.) or a severe reactive hypoglycemic reaction that we sometimes refer to as a "crash and burn" curve because the down slope on the glucose curve is almost vertical. Concurrent PMS can make this a very perplexing situation. Do a pulse test to eliminate allergies and a six-hour GTT.

Treatment should include avoidance of caffeine and sugar in all forms (even the hidden ones, such as fruit, juices, processed sugar, and candy). Take chromium and vanadium 200 - 300 mcg/day, B6 100 mg tid, B3 450 mg tid as time-release tablets, B1, B2, and B5 at the rate of 50 mg tid, L-tryptophan 10 grams tid, calcium 2000 mg/day, and magnesium at 800 mg/day. Betaine HCI 100 - 250 tid before meals and herbs including valerian (Valerian officinalis) can be of value.

ARTERIOSCLEROSIS (hardening of the arteries). It's the result of fibrosis of the smooth muscle in the walls of elastic arteries, notably the aorta and coronary, pulmonary, carotid, cerebral, brachial, and femoral arteries. The elevated "lesions" produce eddies which produce lipid and calcium deposits. Magnesium deficiencies produce "malignant calcification" of elastic arteries and are perhaps the cause of arteriosclerosis.

Elevated blood cholesterol is considered to be a significant risk factor for arteriosclerosis. It is of interest that vitamin D is made from cholesterol in our bodies. This becomes significant when we realize that the toxic effect of vitamin D is angiotoxicity. The target tissue of vitamin D toxicity is the elastic arteries and the specific result is fibrosis of the vascular smooth muscle and calcification of the blood vessel wall—fatty deposits soon follow!

Unfortunately, "orthodox" doctors do not give this as much attention as they do heart transplants, and neither does the media. This information would wipe out a medical specialty, so it's kept under wraps.

Symptoms of arteriosclerosis include angina, headaches, loss of memory, breathlessness, leg cramps ("claudication") in the early stages, and death from stroke and thrombotic-type heart attack in the final stages.

Treatment includes IV chelation with EDTA and H202, oral chelation, oral supplementation with vitamin/mineral supplements that include 800 mg magnesium, and the complete spectrum of plant-derived colloidal minerals. In addition to the baseline nutritional supplements, add vitamin C to bowel tolerance, exercise (to increase the caliber of your arteries), and follow a high fiber, low in animal fat diet. Also supplement with essential fatty acids including salmon oil and flaxseed oil 5 gm tid. Useful herbs include artichoke (Cynara scolymus), bears garlic (Allium ursinum), European mistletoe (Viscum album), cayenne pepper, and garlic (Allium sativum).

ARTHRITIS (rheumatism). This is a devastating

degenerative disease of the joints. Symptoms of joint noise, joint pain, swelling, and deformative changes are typical. The cause of arthritis is listed as unknown by "orthodox" medicine, and the treatment is "take two aspirins a day and call me in the morning." In other words, just learn to live with it.

Prednisone, a synthetic form of cortisone, is used to treat symptoms. In fact, osteoarthritis and degenerative arthritis are a complex of nutritional deficiencies. In the case of rheumatoid arthritis, a chronic infection with a Mycoplasma spp. is the overt cause. Again, if the truth were released, the "orthodox" doctors would lose an entire specialty in short order, so they keep it a secret.

A dietary calcium/phosphorus ratio of 2:1 is ideal yet impossible to attain in an unsupplemented diet. A vegetarian diet gets close but is complicated by "phytates" (a natural chelating substance found in plants) which makes even supplemented calcium unavailable. The calcium/phosphorus ratios of food items is consistent:

Food	Calcium	Phosphorous
Grain	1	8
Red meat	1	12
Organ meat (liver, kidney)	1	44
Fish	1	12
Carbonated drinks	1	8

You can easily see that none of the calcium/phosphorus ratios of the basic foods are anywhere near correct. These increase the calcium loss from the body including the bones and teeth. The more meat you eat, the more calcium supplementation you need. It is quite simple. Veterinarians know this, but they suppose that "orthodox" physicians believe that if a truth will wipe out a medical specialty, it must be ignored or kept a secret!

Treatment of arthritis should include calcium at 2000 mg/day and more if you eat meat two or three times per day. Also take magnesium at 800 - 1000 mg/day, and cartilage (collagen, glucosamine sulfate, and chondroitin sulfate) at 1000 mg tid For rheumatoid arthritis, add tetracyline or minocycline at the low dose acne therapy level daily for one year, or oral food grade $H2O2$ to deal with the Mycoplatsma infection. Intervenous chelation with EDTA and $H2O2$ is very helpful. Take Vitamin C to bowel tolerance, B6 100 mg bid, B3 450 mg bid as time-release capsules. Take Vitamin E at 1000 IU/day. Copper at 2 mg/day (may be absorbed from a copper bracelet), selenium 300 mcg/day, zinc 50 mg tid Plant-derived colloidal minerals are 98% absorbable and give excellent results.

Rotation elimination diets can help when food allergies aggravate or precipitate symptoms. Dr. Wallach's Bone & Joint Pack is an easy formula that can be taken at home that will economically provide all the necessary raw materials to rebuild cartilage, joint capsules, and bone. Autoimmune urine therapy is very useful for all types of arthritis, especially those aggravated by food allergies. DMSO or pain gels are useful in reducing inflammation and pain when applied topically. Herbs including licorice (Glycyrrhiza glabra), poison ivy (Rhus toxicodendron), and alfalfa (powder or sprouts) are useful adjuncts to arthritis treatment programs.

B

BACKACHE This is usually a muscle strain from overwork and/or a "subluxation" (a misalignment of vertebrae) resulting from a fall, osteoporosis, arthritis, bone spurs and calcium deposits, auto accident (whiplash), or improper lifting technique. On occasion, a serious case of constipation will cause a backache from impacted stool or pressure from gas. Eighty-five percent of adult Americans get back problems. Plant-derived colloidal minerals in the form of Dr. Wallach's Bone & Joint Pack have been reported to rebuild cartilage, bones, tendons, and ligaments, thus relieving back problems without surgery.

Prevention includes proper lifting (keep a straight back and bend your knees), strengthening exercises, proper nutrition including calcium (2000 mg) and magnesium (800 mg), high fiber diets, and eight glasses of water per day.

Treatment includes massage, chiropractic, hydrotherapy, Dr. Wallach's Bone & Joint Pack, and poultices of herbs including comfrey (Symphytum officinale) and arnica (Arnica montana).

BAD BREATH (halitosis). This requires basic care. Use a good anti-tartar toothpaste, hydrogen peroxide tooth gel, floss upon awakening and after meals, use a hydrogen peroxide mouthwash, you may use parsley after each meal, and zinc at 50 mg tid Digestive enzymes with betaine HCl may be useful.

BENIGN PROSTATIC HYPERPLASIA This is perhaps the most common infirmity of aging in the human male. More than 500,000 American males (85% over the age of 50) are afflicted each year. As the prostate enlarges with age (usually the result of a zinc deficiency), the tight outer capsule prevents the gland from expanding outwardly so it squeezes down on the neck of the bladder, thus producing the well-recognized symptoms of "frequency" and "urgency" in urination. The prostate is an internal gland that can be "palpated" (felt) with the gloved finger. If you are going to do this exam yourself, it is important to examine the prostate monthly like a woman examines her breasts monthly. The normal prostate is firm like an orange and about the size of a walnut. It is found at a depth in the rectum that is just comfortably in reach for the average length index finger.

Benign prostatic hypertrophy produces a uniform enlargement that may be hard in "acute" enlargement or "boggy" in chronic enlargement. Tumors, either benign or malignant, tend to be irregular and nodular. PSA (Prostate Specific Antigen) may be elevated.

Benign prostatic hypertrophy is treated with zinc at 50 mg tid, essential fatty acids as flaxseed oil at 9 grams per day, high-fiber diets including pumpkin seeds and alfalfa, 300,000 IU vitamin A as beta carotene per day, vitamin C to bowel tolerance, chlorophyll (the best source is alfalfa), amino acids (glycine, alanine, and glutamic acid) at five grams each daily for 90 days, hydrogen peroxide (20 drops per ounce of aloe juice) at 1 ounce bid, unsweetened cranberry juice at two pints per day, herbs including saw pawlmetto (Sarenoa serrulata), and selenium at 250 mcg tid

BELL'S PALSY This is the sudden drooping of one side of the face due to an inflammation, swelling, or squeezing (the result of osteoporosis) of the facial nerve (the seventh cranial nerve as it passes through the skull). Bell's palsy is often mistaken for a stroke because of the sudden onset. Numbness and partial or total loss of muscular control on the affected side of the face are the typical signs and symptoms. Treated properly, there can be as much as an 80% chance of significant recovery.

Treatment is B12 at 1000 mcg/day for a total of 20,000 mcg, calcium/magnesium at 2,000 mg and 800 mg per day, essential fatty acids at 5 gm tid, and American ginseng (Panax quinquefolius). Colloidal minerals are useful. Treat for osteoporosis with Dr. Wallach's Bone & Joint Pack.

BLEEDING GUMS This is an early warning for several problems including vitamin C deficiency (scurvy), calcium deficiency (or bad calcium/phosphorus ratio—osteoporosis), receding gums (the gums recede because of underlying bone loss), or vitamin E deficiency.

Treatment should include vitamin C to bowel tolerance, vitamin E at 800 IU/day, correct dietary calcium/phosphorus ratio with supplemental calcium/magnesium at 2,000 mg and 800 mg, herbal therapy including mouthwash with alpine ragworth (Senecio fuchsii), and mouthwash with aloe/hydrogen peroxide or colloidal silver.

BLOATING (gastric). This is the accumulation of gas in the stomach. Normally, the stomach is sterile because of the acid environment. However, when hypochlorhydria (low stomach acid) occurs, bacteria and yeast from the small intestine migrates up into the stomach. The bacteria in the stomach now "ferments" carbohydrates and sugars that are eaten and produce gas or "bloat."

Treatment of "blech, burp, and bloat" includes oral hydrogen peroxide (20 drops/ounces of liquid to dilute the hydrogen peroxide) at 1 ounce bid, colloidal minerals and betaine HCl, and pancreatic enzymes at 75-200 mg tid 5 minutes before meals.

BOILS (carbuncles, abscesses). These are usually caused by a "staph" infection of the skin and hair follicles. Boils can occur at a site of irritation. Usually, they occur at the neck near a collar line. The tender pus-filled "boil" can be brought to a head by poultices of 3% boric acid and opened with a blade.

Treatment includes flushing the boil with sand sagebrush (Artemisa fififolia), enchinacea (Echinacea angustifolia) and/or hydrogen peroxide, vitamin C at bowel tolerance, vitamin A at 300,000 IU/day as beta carotene, and zinc 50 mg tid. Antibiotic ointment may be considered if new boils appear until the vitamins and minerals begin to take effect. Don't forget the baseline supplements.

BONE PAIN (including "spurs," calcium deposits, Osgood-Slaughter, Legg-Perthes). This can be immobilizing and crippling. Bone pain can be part of the "growing pains," especially at the joints or the insertions of tendons into bones (which is where spurs occur). Bone pain is a self-diagnosing problem. If it persists, x-rays should be taken to confirm diagnosis of fracture, arthritis, spurs, or rule out the more severe problem of primary or metastatic bone cancer.

Treatment of bone pain and spurs includes Dr. Wallach's Bone & Joint Pack, vitamin C to bowel tolerance, vitamin E at 800-1,200 IU/day, and magnesium at 500 mg tid for as long as one to two years. Correct the calcium/phosphorus ratio with calcium at 2,000 mg/day and reduce meat intake. Herbs including comfrey (Symphytum officinale) may be helpful. Plant-derived colloidal minerals have reversed spurs and calcium deposits without surgery by remodeling the bone.

BRITTLE NAILS This is a common ailment, especially in vegetarians, teenagers, pregnant women, and individuals with food allergies. The causes of brittle nails are malabsorption or deficiencies of essential fatty acids, amino acids (low protein/vegetarian diets), collagen, keratin, calcium, iron, or zinc.

Treatment of brittle nails includes dealing with food allergies to improve absorption, gelatin (unflavored and unsweetened or diabetic brands), essential fatty acids at 5 gm tid, vitamin E at 800-1,200 IU/day, the baseline supplementation, and betaine HCl and pancreatic enzymes at 75-200 mg each tid 15 minutes before meals. To diagnose food allergies, use the pulse test--it's cheap and accurate.

BRONCHITIS (grippe, catarrh, chest colds). This can be caused by viral or bacterial infections. Allergies, both food and inhalant, will aggravate bronchitis as will essential fatty acid, magnesium, and manganese deficiencies. If bronchitis persists after treatment for five to ten days, consider cystic fibrosis in children and lung cancer in adults. X-rays will be necessary to determine diagnosis of chronic processes.

Treatment includes steam vaporizers at night, essential fatty acids at 5 gm tid, digestive enzymes and betaine HCl at 75-200 mg each, vitamin C to bowel tolerance, Vitamin A at 300,000 IU as beta carotene, coltsfoot (Tussilago farfara), cowslip (Primula veris), eucalptus (Eucalyptus globulus) as a poultice/chest rub and/or placed in vaporizer, Irish moss (Chondrus crispus), pansy (Viola tricolor), pleurisy root (Asclepias tuberose), and holly hock (Althaea rosea).

BRUISES This is the result of a bump or a blow that ruptures blood vessels and releases blood into the surrounding tissue including the skin. The fragility (tenderness) of capillaries can result from overdoses of blood thinners, copper deficiency, or vitamin K, vitamin C, or vitamin E deficiencies.

Treatment includes vitamin C to bowel tolerance, vitamin E at 800-1,200 IU per day, vitamin K at 30 mcg per day, and pancreatic enzymes at 200 mg tid between meals. Take enzymes between meals so they get into your bloodstream and dissolve blood clots. Take DMSO topically, pain gel, and herbs including arnica (Arnica montana), marigold (Calendula officinalis), witch hazel (Hamaelis virginiana), and yellow sweet clover (Metilotus officinalis).

BRUXISM (teeth grinding). This is the clenching or grinding of teeth. Bruxism usually occurs during sleep and is, therefore, often overlooked until wear of the dental enamel is observed. Bruxism can be the result of food allergies (use the pulse test to find out; sugar, milk, and wheat tend to be the offenders), hypoglycemia (bed-wetting and nightmares may occur with bruxism if hypoglycemia is involved), or deficiencies of calcium, magnesium, and/or B6.

Treatment includes avoidance or rotation of offending food and elimination of sugar from the diet especially before bed. Also, take calcium and magnesium at 2,000 mg and 1,000 mg per day and B6 at 50 mg tid

BURSITIS This is an inflammation of bursal sacs that cushion tendons as they pass over joints (i.e., shoulder, "housemaid's knee," "miner's elbow," and "bunions"). Overwork of an out-of-shape joint can bring on a flare up. Don't forget the baseline vitamins and minerals as a preventative along with moderate exercise.

Treatment of bursitis includes topical pain gels, DMSO, or liniments with eucalyptus to bring more circulation to the area and remove swelling (which is the source of bursitis pain). Oral support includes B12 at 1,000 mcg/day, vitamin C to bowel tolerance, bioflavonoids 1,200 mg/day, rutin 50 mg and 1,000 mg per day respectively, gelatin, cartilage 5 gm tid and alfalfa. Be sure to include Dr. Wallach's Bone & Joint Pack in your bursitis treatment program

CALCULUS (tartar). This is a buildup of calcium carbonate on the tooth, usually at the gingival junction where the gum attaches to the tooth. The source of the calcium is the patient's own bony calcium which is being lost in the saliva. That's why tartar is worst on the back of the lower incisors. When this happens, you may need more magnesium to hold calcium in the bones and correct a severe dietary calcium/phosphorus ratio problem. Reduce red meat, soft drinks, and any other major source of phosphorus in the diet. The use of hydrogen peroxide tooth gels and anti-tartar toothpastes will help reduce existing tarter and prevent build up.

Treatment of calculus and tartar includes flossing, use of a dental pick that you can purchase from a pharmacy to pop off large "plates" of hardened material from the back of, and between, teeth, and use of a firm toothbrush and hydrogen peroxide tooth gels and tartar control toothpaste. Treat for osteoporosis with Dr. Wallach's Bone & Joint Pack.

CATARACTS These are caused by changes in the eye lens, which makes them opaque and unable to transmit light to the retina of the eye. Cataracts are easily diagnosed with the ophthalmoscope in a darkened examining room. Severe mature cataracts are snow white and opaque like mothballs and are easily seen with the unaided eye through the pupil of the eye. Cataracts are the most common cause of blindness in older people and should be dealt with aggressively and without delay.

Treatment of cataracts includes avoiding fried food and margarine, the baseline vitamin/mineral supplement plus vitamin E at 2,000 IU/day, vitamin C to bowel tolerance, B1, B2, B3, B5, and B6 at 50 mg bid, inositol at 150 mg/day, selenium at 250 mcg/day, zinc at 25 tid, bioflavonoids at 300 mg., glycerine at 200 mg, 1-glutamine at 200 mg, 1-arginine at 300 mg/day, 1-cysteine at 400 mg/day, and glutathione at 40 mg/day. If diabetes or hypoglycemia is present, chromium and vanadium at 250 mcg tid should be added.

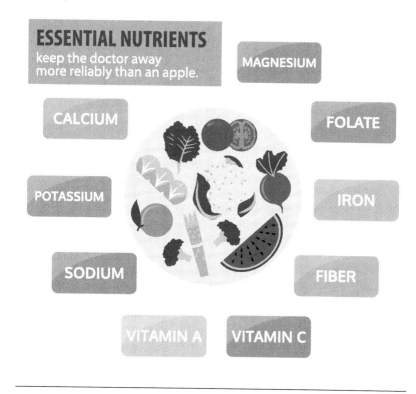

What Are Essential Nutrients?

Every human being who dies of natural causes dies of a nutritional deficiency disease. We like to believe that no one can die of a nutritional deficiency in America. Doctors, medical experts, bureaucrats, and professors all like to say that there's no evidence that you can prevent and cure disease with vitamins and minerals.

But we know **THE TRUTH.**

You might not have known how to treat all of the diseases you just read about in The ABCs of Diseases and Their Cures section of this book and the A to Z section found in my book, Dead Doctors Don't Lie. But we're all familiar with the more obvious examples of what causes diseases like scurvy, rickets, goiter, anemia, and more.

You've heard this before, haven't you?

> **SCURVY.** That's what you get when you lack vitamin C.
>
> **RICKETS.** That's what happens when you lack vitamin D.
>
> **GOITER.** You can prevent and cure goiter with iodine, copper, and selenium.
>
> **ANEMIA.** You can prevent it, and cure it, with iron, copper, folic acid, and Vitamin B12.

And what about beriberi with congestive heart failure? Do you know you can cure that with thiamine or vitamin B1?

And what about pellagra, and schizophrenia, diarrhea, and all the skin diseases that go along with pellagra? Did you know that you can prevent and cure that with vitamin B3 or niacin?

That's right. You probably have heard all of this before. In fact, you knew about essential nutrients all along. You just didn't know they had a name.

The essential nutrients are called the essential nutrients because, if you don't have enough of them, you get diseases. It's simple.

> **ESSENTIAL NUTRIENTS KEEP THE DOCTOR AWAY MORE RELIABLY THAN AN APPLE.**

But the good news is that, if you get the disease, and then you take the nutrient, the disease goes away.

So What's the Argument?

With scurvy, rickets, goiter, anemia, beriberi, and pellagra, the cures are probably obvious to everyone. So where's the argument to be made against using essential nutrients to treat these diseases?

There isn't a reasonable argument to be made. Any expert who makes the claim that you can't prevent and cure diseases with vitamins and minerals is a fool, and you don't want to have a fool for a doctor.

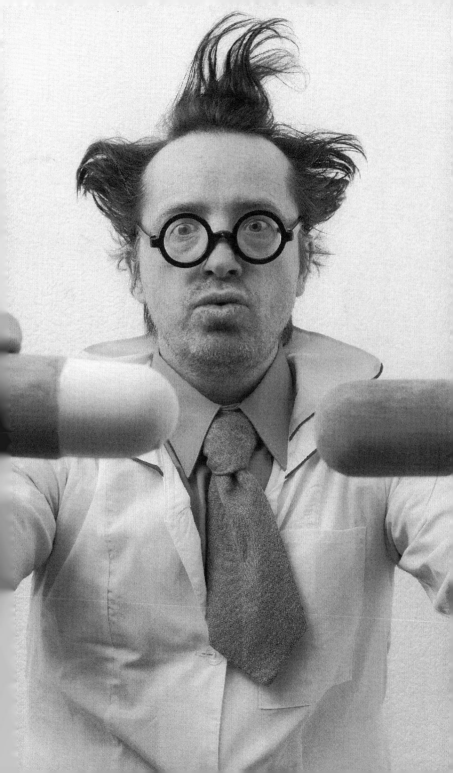

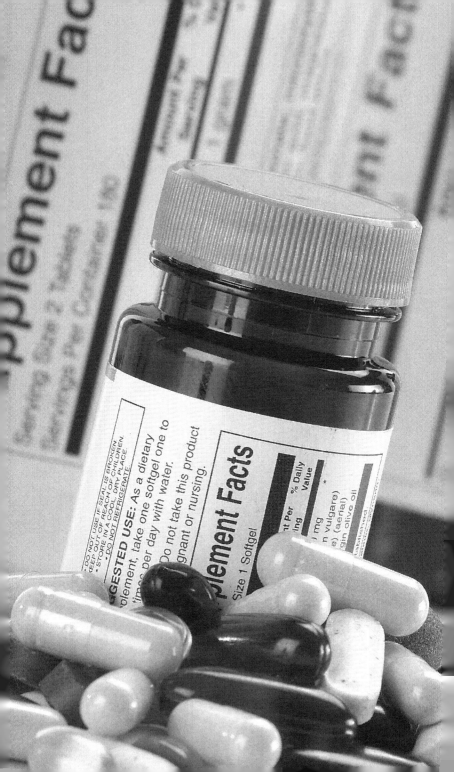

CHAPTER 3

WHY DO WE NEED SUPPLEMENTS?

WHAT TO EXPECT

In October 2002, a World Health Organization study found that life expectancy closely mirrors dietary factors. Nearly one-third of early death and disability stems from nutritional or dietary causes, including too little food in the poorest countries and the wrong kind of food in the richest countries.

This was the most profound observation the study made: inadequate intake of three key micronutrients, zinc, iron, and Vitamin A, is responsible for an unexpectedly high burden of disease.

There are ninety essential nutrients. The study didn't even look at the other eighty-seven.

Finally, forty years later, the World Health Organization came to the same conclusion that I did forty years earlier. So I feel pretty good about that.

There are all of these essential nutrients, and there are two reasons why they're called essential nutrients. Number one, our bodies cannot manufacture them, and so we must consume them every day, either as food or as supplements. Number two, if you're missing some of them, you will get some horrible collection of diseases, many of which are life threatening.

THAT'S WHY THEY'RE CALLED ESSENTIAL NUTRIENTS.

What Are Minerals?

Of all the essential nutrients, the ones I'd like to focus on here are minerals, because minerals make up two-thirds of the essential nutrients.

Our food plants, which are grains, vegetables, fruits, and nuts, cannot manufacture minerals. They can manufacture vitamins, amino acids, and fatty acids. We know that. But no plant can manufacture a mineral. Nutritional minerals do not occur in a uniform crust around the Earth. Nutritional minerals occur in veins just like chocolate in chocolate ripple ice cream, or like gold and silver. The odds of getting all the essential nutrients and all the essential minerals just by eating well is zero. Here's why.

In the same field, on one farm, for instance, row number one of a certain crop might have three essential minerals. Row number five might have zero. Row number ten might have eight. Row number fifteen might have twenty. Row number twenty might have zero. Row number twenty-five might have zero. Row number thirty might have sixteen. So the minerals you're getting depends on which row in the field your tomato, corn, soybeans, or wheat came from. Since there is a vast difference in mineral content in different rows or different parts of one field, you can imagine the difference in different fields in different parts of the same valley and then different valleys in the same state and then different countries, etc. You have no idea when you are picking up produce at the local market, which minerals were absorbed by each particular carrot or orange.

We Are Not Carrots

To be happy, most plants only need about nine minerals. Humans need sixty minerals. So the plants are happy, and when you look at them, you think, "Wow, this is a really good looking carrot." It has nine minerals. But what about the other fifty-one?

It doesn't make sense to throw your life away, or to sacrifice part of your longevity or your health, because of what may or

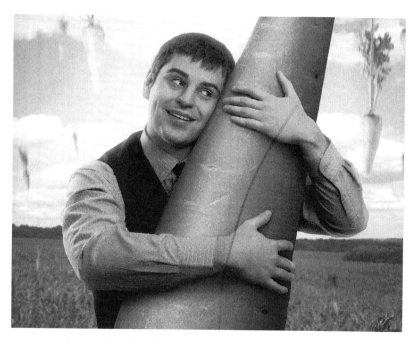

may not be in the food. You can't tell by looking at the carrot. As long as it's getting its nine minerals, it's happy. But that isn't good enough, and you shouldn't bet your life on that carrot.

Soil Depletion

And then there's another problem: soil depletion. Much of the world's soil is seriously depleted. Healthy crops depend on healthy soil. But nearly forty percent of the land used for agriculture is seriously degraded which means it doesn't have these nutrients in it anymore.

African soils over the last hundred years (as of 1992) had been depleted, and its fertility by 74%; Asia by 73%; Australia by 55%; Europe by 72%; South American by 76%; and the United States and North America by 85%. And since 1992, it has only become worse.

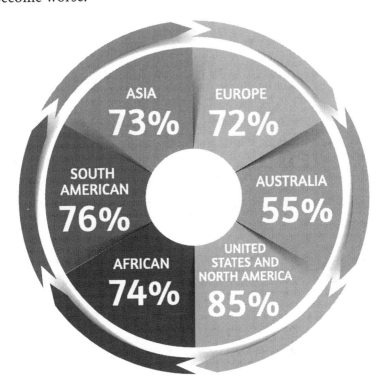

There's been a 53% decrease in the calcium values, a 38% drop in vitamin A, and a 48% drop in riboflavin, broccoli, cabbage, carrots, cauliflower, collards, kale, mustard greens, onion, parsley, turnip greens, watercress, and so forth. If you're not putting the essential minerals in the soil that the plant needs, their ability to manufacture vitamins begins to drop. Today, there's only about 8% protein in our wheat. In 1900, there was 23%.

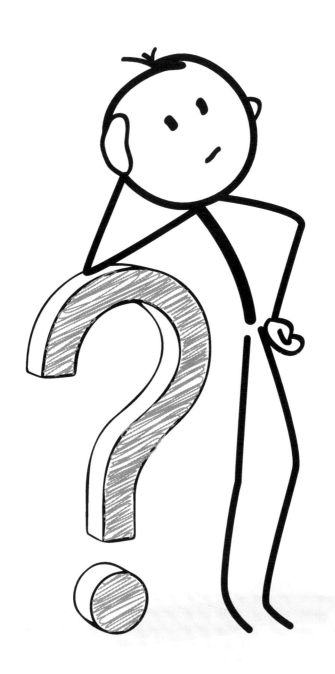

CHAPTER 4

WHAT DOES LONGEVITY LOOK LIKE?

Do You Want to Live to Be 100?

My goal, as a physician, was to enable patients to live to be 100 instead of only 75. In 1978, a certain percentage of my patients would say, "I don't think I'd want to live to be 100." I'd say, "Why wouldn't you want to live to be 100?" They'd answer me, "Well, I don't want to wind up in a nursing home." I thought that was a reasonable concern, so I began to collect research on those who had lived to be 100 that would satisfy me that I was doing the right thing to help my patients live to be 100.

Studies have shown that people who don't listen to their doctors are more likely to live to be 100 than those who do follow their doctors' advice. They eat butter, salt, cheese, chicken skin, and eggs, and the only exercise they get when they came home from work is to fall asleep on the couch.

Researchers were flabbergasted. They couldn't figure out why people who were doing all the wrong things were living so long. Obviously, people were getting inappropriate advice from their doctors.

An Animal Model for Longevity

So what would it take to live to be 100? I looked for an animal model first. Doing some research, I ran into some stuff that was published in 1863. I read something about how to cure corpulence, which is an old-fashioned word for obesity. The author talked about a low-carb diet, like the Atkins diet. And then, in 1935, a guy who had been doing all this research in the 1920s, Clive M. McKay, came out with his landmark article.

His article was about an experiment he did with rats. They were divided into three groups. He gave group number one a rat pellet that contained the most nutritious foods known about in that day, and these rats lived an average of two years. That was exciting, because laboratory rats ordinarily were given rolled oats, carrots, and cabbage, and they might live eleven months after they were weaned. So it was really good to find a food you could give rats to make them live for two years.

He then gave the second group the same basic pellet as the first group. So he kept the vitamins and the minerals the same, but he cut the carbohydrate calories by thirty percent. They lived to be an average of three years old, which was fifty percent longer than ordinary laboratory rats.

Finally, McKay cut the carbohydrate calories by sixty percent for group number three. He kept the vitamins and the minerals the same. They lived twice as long: four years!

But it wasn't just the carbohydrate calories, because when they did the study again with spiders, beetles, worms, pigeons, and all kinds of animals, they found out that it was the density of the vitamins and the minerals per remaining carbohydrate calorie. That was the basic reason, because he had always kept the vitamins and minerals the same when he dropped the calories. He didn't just drop the percentage of food. He dropped only the carbohydrate calories, keeping everything else the same. So in group number three, there was three times the amount of vitamins and minerals per carbohydrate calorie than there was in group number one. That made all the difference.

The Human Model for Longevity

Now that I had an animal model for longevity, I began to look for a human model. I ran into a person whose name you may know: Art Linkletter. He was a funny comedian who could tell great stories without using dirty words—I put Milton Berle, Jack Benny, and Art Linkletter into the same category—who lived to be 97 years old.

He was inspired by a novel called Lost Horizon, which was written by James Hilton. A utopian adventure novel, it was where the concept of Shangri-La originated. Linkletter, after reading the book, decided that he wanted to live to be 100. Lost Horizon was about a people called the Hunzas from the northeast of Pakistan which is a third-world country. Linkletter hired Dr. Allen E. Banik, an eye doctor who was an amateur farmer, and he funded him to go there for six months during the growing season and find out what their secret was for living to be 100. Dr. Banik wrote a book called *The Fabulous Health and Youth Wonderland of the World*.

It was obvious from Dr. Banik's book that he hadn't read Clive McKay's material on rats. He was just making a lot of observations and not reaching conclusions, but he was a good observer. One of the things he observed is that these people had no electricity, no indoor plumbing, no hospitals, no pharmacies, no clinics, and no doctors. They just used home remedies like herbs and massage therapy. Yet they were the healthiest, long-lived people on Earth. They came from a little-known mountain range called the Karakoram Mountains, about 800 miles east of the Himalayas.

One of the things that Dr. Banik observed was that they would irrigate with water that was grey and opaque and had lots of silt in it from the glacier grinding up the mountain rocks. They would irrigate with this glacial water full of this finely ground up rock silt, about the same particle size as talc, and it contained over sixteen minerals. As the water percolated down into their fields and gardens, it left a half inch to an inch of this grey silt on top of the soil. And, before it dried, they would run out with their hoes and their rakes, and they would mix this silt into their soil. These people lived 19,500 feet above sea level. At that level, you can't grow corn, rice, and potatoes. Ninety-nine percent of the original valley was bare rock. That means the indigenous plant life of the Hunza Valley was rather limited.

They could grow wheat, rye, and barley. But because of the short growing season, their yields were small. The only carbohydrate they ate during the day was a tiny tortilla, a little round, flat bread. The majority of their food was goat, lamb, mutton, camel, yak, rabbits, chickens, and eggs. They were too high up for fish. They cooked in butter (and also put it in their tea). They used milk, cheese, and yogurt, and that was it. If they had a little garden, they'd grow cabbage, tomatoes, and little else. They breast-fed their children until they were between two and four years old. They would also put wood ashes from their fires into their gardens.

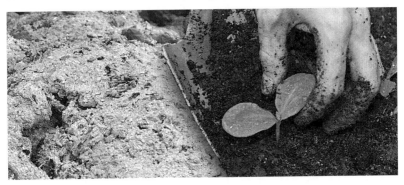

How many of you have ever put wood ashes from your fireplace into your garden?

This is an old European and Asian custom. Putting wood ashes into your garden increases the yield and makes the food taste better.

Well, it turns out that wood ashes are the minerals that are left when you burn away the carbon in the wood.

Plants, including wild forms and crops such as grains, vegetables, fruits, and nuts, take up these inorganic metallic colloids and convert them into intracellular (within the cell), organically bound plant colloids. These organic plant colloids are the form of minerals found in and used by all living cells of plants, animals, and humans. It is the eating of the plants rich in organic colloidal minerals that is the secret of health and longevity.

Fourteen Hunza Secrets

Here are the 14 Hunza practices that contributed to their longevity:

1. The basic diet consisted of grains (whole grain and sprouted), vegetables (raw or steamed), fruits (fruits are dried and reconstituted in water or diced and served in gelatin from goat and mutton tendon and cartilage). Meat was consumed at two or four pounds per person, per week. Mutton, goat, yak, beef, poultry, brain, kidney, and liver were eaten as available. Dairy, including whole milk, buttermilk, yogurt, cheese, and butter were staples. A grape wine known as Pani was consumed daily. Contrary to popular belief, the Hunzas were definitely not vegetarians!

2. Their farm soils were maintained by organic agricultural practices, which means that which was taken from the soil was returned to the soil. Composting, plant debris, and animal manure was turned back into the soil.
3. All Hunzas worked 12 hours each day, seven days each week--for them, there is no Sabbath, sick leave, vacation days, or maternity leave. Work doesn't appear to kill anyone.
4. Fat sources included whole milk, butter, ghee, apricot oil, and animal fats.
5. There was a total absence of additives, preservatives, and chemicals in their air, food, and water.
6. They consumed salt daily by adding chunks of rock salt to their tea, and in cooking vegetables and meat.
7. They used no agricultural sprays or chemicals of any kind.
8. All children were breast fed for two (girls) to four (boys) years. Traditionally, there were no vaccines or antibiotics. There were few, if any, birth defects recorded except for two hermaphrodites or mukhanas in the 2,300 years of recorded Hunza history.
9. All grains, vegetables, and fruits were dried for storage by use of the sun.
10. Native herbs were used for medicine, seasoning, and food. There were no western-style hospitals or doctors in Hunza. Part of their longevity success was due to the avoidance of injury and death found in industrial nations at the hands of high-tech health practioners.
11. Glacial milk was the exclusive water source used for drinking and irrigation purposes. The fields were

flooded with glacial milk and, when the water soaks into the soil, a thick layer of mineral silt or "rock flour" was left on top of the soil. The silt was plowed into the soil before planting. The crops converted the metallic rock flour into colloidal mineral rich crops. As a result of regular consumption of the essential minerals, the people were relatively disease free and lived well past a hundred.

12. Apricot oil was used for cooking along with ghee (clarified butter) and yak, beef, mutton, or goat fat (tallow).
13. Whole grains were used exclusively—no processed or white flours.
14. The Hunza ate 1,800 to 2,000 calories each day

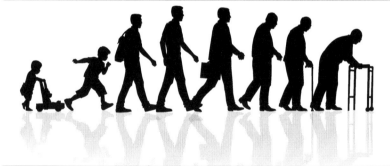

What We Know About the Human Model

So now I had not only an animal model and a human model, but we know these facts about the human model. They had a renewable source of minerals in their food. They were on a low carbohydrate diet. And that explained why they lived to be a ripe old age.

That explained why, although they were very much members of our species, they were a very select subgroup of our species. They were centenarians.

What Are Centenarians?

No, the centenarians aren't an alien race from a new science fiction television series or film. They're human beings just like you and I…except they've lived longer than most of us.

Centenarians are people who have lived to be at least a hundred years old.

They may not be highly educated, although there's nothing to stop them from having impressive high school diplomas, college degrees, or even graduate degrees or doctorates.

They may not be wealthy (although, certainly, they can amass fortunes).

They may not be famous. Then again, they might be well known for something.

There's no particular requirement they be good looking, but there's nothing to stop them from being attractive or glamorous.

In fact, they may be no different from your neighbors. They might even be your neighbors.

Centenarians simply are those people who have achieved longevity. Let's meet some of them.

Meet the Centenarians!

To meet the centenarians, I began to collect birth announcements and obituaries of people who lived to be 100. I wanted to see what happened to people when they reached that achievement and joined that group. What I found surprised even me, and I had an open mind! These were not the people who come to mind when you think of "little old men" or "little old women."

Centenarians Are Amazing!

HERE ARE JUST A FEW OF THEM.

Ralph Charles, from Somerset, Ohio, was the subject of a local newspaper story when he turned 100 in October of 1999. The fascinating thing was that, at age 100, he was still piloting charter airline flights and carrying paying passengers around the central part of the United States. He used his single engine Aeronca Defender aircraft. He didn't have any restrictions on his license. When you look at the photograph that accompanies the newspaper article, he doesn't look like what you'd expect a decrepit 100-year old to look like. To me, he appears to be very vibrant. He looks as if he's in his late 70s or early 80s. He's 100 years old, at the time of the publication of that newspaper story, and he's still flying a plane. He doesn't have Alzheimer's disease or any type of dementia. He doesn't get up into the sky and ask his passengers where he's supposed to be going. But he didn't have those problems, obviously.

Connie Douglas Reeves turned 101 in September of 2002. At that age, she was inducted in the National Cowgirl Hall of Fame. Her personal motto was: Always saddle your own horse. To me, she looks like one of those feisty people who wouldn't listen to a doctor. In the newspaper photo, she has her thumbs in her belt, she has her shoulders back, and she has her chin jutting out. You can just imagine a doctor saying to her, "Look, Connie, you're 101-years old now. It's time to give up salt. We have to worry about your blood pressure. It's time to give up eggs and butter. We have to worry about your cholesterol." And she's going to say, "No way, mister! That isn't happening. I've been eating salt, eggs, and butter since before you were born, and I'm not going to give that up!" You can almost hear that conversation as you look at her photograph. She is definitely not a shrinking violet!

In May of 2001, Harold Stilson from Deer Beach, Florida went out and played golf for his 101st birthday, and he hit his sixth hole in one! Now, to do that, you have to have a strong grip, you have to be able to see 108 yards, you have to have good eye to hand coordination, you have to have a good memory or else you'd start to swing your golf club and forget what you're doing. You'd be saying, "What was I doing? Was I swinging a baseball bat?" You can see, from his picture in the newspaper, that he's color coordinated in the way he dresses. It doesn't get any better than that for 101 years old.

Then there's Antonio Todde from Tiana, in the province of Nuoro, Sardinia, a rural community. In January 2001, he turned 112. He attributed his longevity to drinking one glass of red wine each day. There's a certain amount of validity to that, because in the red wine, there were these antioxidants that we know reduce your risk of heart disease and cancer. But you can get the same antioxidants in fruits and vegetables. You don't necessarily need to drink the wine. It doesn't seem to matter what you eat, as long as you keep your carbohydrates down, and the vitamins and minerals up. That seems to be the common thread between all centenarians.

Dorah Ramothibe from Vosloorus, South Africa. was born in 1881 and, in 1995, she turned 114. When she was asked what she attributed her health and longevity to, she said she ate locusts. "You know about grasshoppers, don't you?" she asked. She also ate pumpkin seeds, tortoise meat, wild herbs, dried fruit, and drank a cup of coffee each day. She didn't mention bread, potatoes, rice, or corn. The only carbohydrate in her diet might have been a little bit of that dried fruit. She got her protein from the locusts and the tortoise meat. She got her essential fatty acids from the pumpkin seeds, and if she ate the herbs when they were fresh, she got her vitamin C, folic acid, and beta carotene from them.

On February 6, 2003, Mattie Owens, a former field hand, maid, homemaker, and mother of four passed away at 119. She grew up in South Carolina. When she was born, in 1883, her family was working in the cotton field, and she did too. I guarantee she didn't have vaccinations. I guarantee you she didn't have antibiotics. I guarantee you she didn't have three square meals a day. But—because I spent two years in Africa, and I know what they did there with the wood ashes from their cooking fires for their cabbage, tomatoes, and beans, and so forth—I'll bet you her parents put their wood ashes from their cooking fires into the gardens.

And one of my favorite birth announcements goes back to 1875. This was a birth announcement for Jeanne Calment from France. She was documented as being one of the oldest living women at the time. Other women claimed to be older than she was, but they didn't have the paperwork to prove it. Jeanne Calment had the paperwork to prove, to the satisfaction of the Guinness Book of World Records, that on February 21, 1995, she was, in fact, 120 years old. She died in August of 1997 at age 122. She died suddenly, of a stroke. She was up cooking her eggs and singing Frère Jacques. She didn't have Alzheimer's disease. She was mentally alert until the moment she died. She didn't have cardiovascular disease. She didn't have diabetes. She didn't have cancer. She did have rheumatoid arthritis in her hands, as you can see from her picture in the newspaper, but that's pretty good considering she lived to be 122. That's the way to do it.

Sek Yi, a man from Cambodia, also died at age 122. He was a martial arts expert and a tiger hunter. He attributed his longevity (and that of his wife, Long Ouk) to smoking and prayer. That's kind of a strange combination, but it worked for them! And I'm sure he got some minerals from somewhere.

A Brazilian named Maria Etelvina Dos Santos lived to be 124. She died of a stroke. Her birth certificate says, the daughter of African slaves, she was born on July 18, 1878. Do you think she got vaccinations and antibiotics and a list of prescriptions?

Do you think she had three square meals a day? No. She was born in a straw hut caulked with cow dung. She probably led a pretty miserable life as she was growing up. But I guarantee you they put their wood ashes from their cooking fires into their gardens. They didn't have doctors, and they didn't have hospitals and clinics, and they didn't have pharmaceuticals. And yet she lived to be 124.

This man I identify with because I grew up on a cattle farm in Missouri where we raised purebred Angus cattle. Narayan Chaudhuri, too, was a cattle farmer from a little town outside of Katmandu in the Himalayan Mountains. According to his obituary, he never saw a doctor, and he never set foot inside a hospital. He smoked two packs of cigarettes a day for 120 years. He wasn't a vegetarian. Raising cattle, he ate red meat every day. Although he didn't have a birth certificate, he was honored as the oldest man in Nepal. In April of 1998, he died when he was reportedly 141 years old. When he was a young man, he led the first land survey team around Katmandu in 1888.

In July 2015, Evelyn Jones threw out the first pitch at the Mariner's baseball game against the Los Angeles Angels in Safeco Field in Seattle, Washington. A native of Woodinville, Washington, she's been a life-long Mariners fan, and she still hopes to see her team make a World Series game. Don't tell her that she "throws like a girl." At 108 years old, she's earned some respect. As ESPN reported, Evelyn is the oldest person to ever throw out the first pitch at a major league game. The person who previously held that position was Agnes McKee, who tossed a pitch before a Padres game in the summer of 2014 at age 105.

The last centenarian that I want to share with you tells a lot of stories. This is one of my favorite obituaries from January 1995. It's about an Iranian woman named Mazumi Doosti. The obituary says that she died at 161. Now that seems like an outrageous claim, but you have to give a lot of credence to the story because, reportedly, she was survived by six living children ranging in age from 120 to 128. Her oldest son, Gholam, observed that his mother had never visited a doctor, never taken any prescription medications or over-the-counter medications. She only used herbs. They were born up in the mountains of Iran. I guarantee you that she was functional until very close to her death because they don't have nursing homes, and they're not going to find some way to give her IVs to keep her alive. She had to be still able to snap beans, peel carrots, cook, and sing lullabies to her great, great, great grandkids.

> **WE ALL HAVE THESE GENETIC CAPACITIES TO LIVE WELL BEYOND 100.**

We know for a fact that humans can live to be 122 years and 164 days because the Guinness Book of World Records says so.

Eight Model Cultures

There are eight well-known cultures whose peoples routinely live to their maximum genetic potential of 120 to 140 years of age. The fact that all eight cultures are Third World countries is significant and, collectively, they are known as the Agebeaters cultures. No one can argue that these long-lived centenarians from Third World countries do a much better job than we do in reaching their genetic potential for longevity

The longest average longevity held by an industrialized nation is attributed to the Japanese who live on the average to 79.1. On the other hand, the Himalayan Tibetans from the northwest of China, the Hunzakut from the Karakarum Mountains of eastern Pakistan, the Russian Georgians from the Caucus Mountains in western Russia (and their sister cultures of Armenia, Azerbaijian, Abkhazia, and Turkey), the Vilcabamba from the Andes of Ecuador, and the Titicacas of the Andes of Peru are all famous for their high percentage of centenarians.

The Common Good

So what are the eight model cultures of longevity doing right? Here are the six good things they have in common:

1. The communities are found at elevations ranging from 8,500 feet to 14,000 feet in sheltered mountain valleys.
2. Their annual precipitation is less than two inches.
3. Their water source for drinking and irrigation comes from the glacial melt and is known universally as "glacial milk" because the highly mineralized water is an opaque white or gray in color, and because of the presence of an enormous amount of suspended rock flour.
4. There is no heavy industry or modern agriculture to pol

ute their air, water, or food.
5. Only natural fertilizer including animal manure, plant debris, and "glacial milk" is applied to their fields.
6. Western allopathic medicine was not historically available to these cultures, so they were able to avoid stepping on that landmine—blind faith in orthodox doctors of today.

The Scorecard

Experts in longevity, gerontology, and genetics tell us that every one of us has the genetic capability to live well beyond 100. The only reason we don't is because we do too much of the bad stuff, and not enough of the good stuff.

People do live to be 120 to 140 years of age. They do it all the time. Some extraordinary individuals will live to be 150 and 160. The only question is: how can we get there from here without moving near a glacier?

One of the most fascinating things, to me, is that we ask doctors what to do about health and longevity. Now, if doctors knew what they were talking about, that would make sense.

But I'm a scorecard kind of guy, so I'm looking at doctors and saying do they really, really know what they're talking about.

When I taped "Dead Doctors Don't Lie," which came out in 1994, I had a statistic in there from a small survey that said doctors live to be 57.6 (and I rounded it up to 58 to give them the benefit of the doubt). And doctors just went ballistic. They said, "Dr. Wallach, you're lying. We don't live to be 58! We live to be 75, just like everybody else."

Well, even if they lived to be 75, just like everybody else, that wouldn't be too good of a recommendation because, if they're the holders of all knowledge about health, and they follow their own recommendations, they should live to be 85 or 95 or 100. Even still, I showed that they only lived to be 58, far below the 75.

They didn't want to believe me, so they did their own study. It was published 5 years later in 1999, and they found that doctors in America live to be 56. So I missed it by 2 years.

> **IS THERE A DOCTOR IN THE HOUSE?**
> **GOOD! LOCK THE DOOR—QUICKLY!**

So why would we ask people who live to be only 56 on average how to live long, healthy lives? That's because they have convinced us that healthcare is very complicated, and you have to go to school for 14 years to know how to deal with healthcare.

They've convinced Americans this is true. You can't pick up a newspaper, watch TV, surf the web, or listen to the radio without healthcare, Medicare, Medicaid, and all related issues being on the front burner.

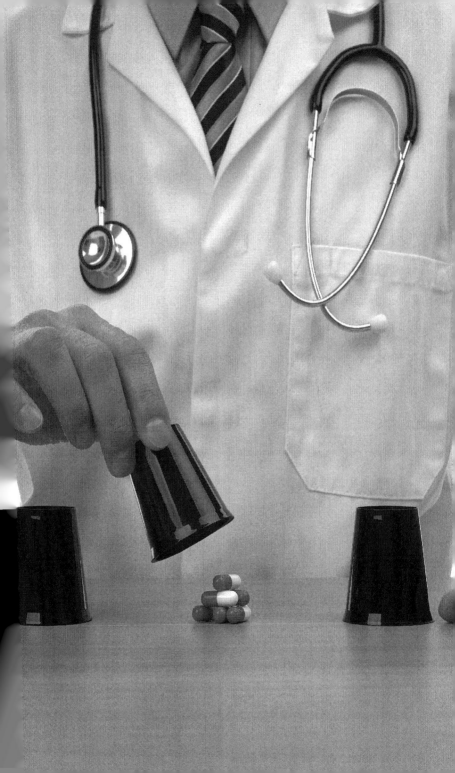

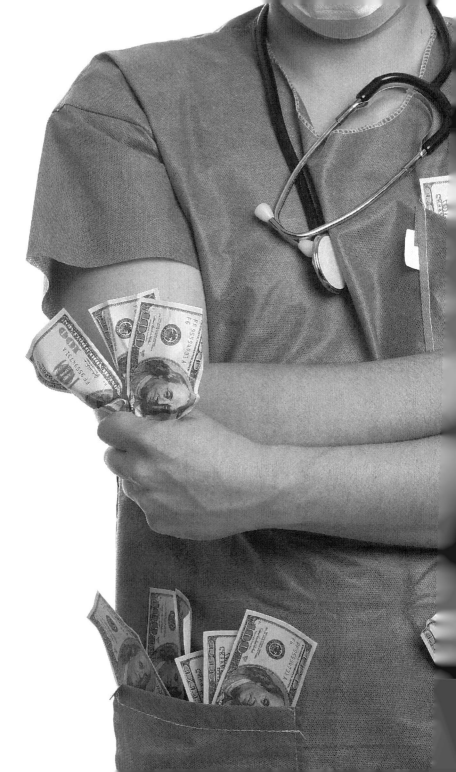

CHAPTER 5

MISPLACED TRUST

The Healthcare Buck

Let's look at more scorecards and see whether we're getting the biggest bang for the buck. Right now, the entire world spends 2.7 trillion dollars each year for healthcare. The U.S. alone spends 1.6 trillion dollars, more than half.

And, yet, in April of 1990, we ranked 17th in longevity. There were 16 other countries whose peoples live longer than we do.

We didn't even rank in the top 10. You have to ask, "Who was number 1, and what did they do differently from us?" The Japanese were number 1. They lived to be 79.1, which was 4.1 years longer than we did.

Ten years later, in June of 2000, they conducted the same study again. The Japanese maintained the number one position. This was our chance to catch up and surpass them with all this money we're spending on healthcare. Right?

But, instead, we dropped from 17th in longevity all the way down to 24th. The Japanese still rank number one today with an average life expectancy of 84.

Maybe we have improved in the last 15 years with all our new modern advances, and more schooled doctors and more prescription drugs? Well, we now actually rank 40th in longevity. You may have heard that in the United States we have the BEST healthcare system in the world. If by BEST, you mean most profitable for doctors and pharmaceutical companies, then I suppose there is some truth to that.

Interestingly, the Japanese were heavy smokers. Sixty-eight percent of the Japanese smoked three to five packs of cigarettes each day.

THEY ARE THE "SMOKINGEST" NATION ON EARTH.

Yet they have 85% less cancer and cardiovascular disease than we do.

Japanese consume 12 to 15 grams of salt every day. That's an entire salt shaker per person. We're supposed to consume approximately 1 gram, or 1,000 milligrams, of salt per day.

We dropped two atomic bombs on the Japanese in World War 2. They've had more radiation per person than any other culture on Earth. Nobody cleaned it up. They've been wallowing in all the radiation in their soil and water and environment since we dropped the bombs on them, and they have 85% less cancer than we do.

> **SO I WANT TO KNOW WHAT THEY KNOW.**

In all this adversity, they're still living longer than we are. And they're healthier than we are.

You don't have to be a genius to figure out we're not getting the bang for the healthcare buck. Maybe the medication we're getting isn't doing any good. Maybe the advice we're getting is not the best. No matter what the doctors tell us, we're going in the wrong direction. They can't deny the facts, and neither can we.

There are 250,000 drugs that doctors have to treat people in America, and there are new ones coming out all the time. They're always bragging about how many billions of dollars they spend on research during the course of a year to find new drugs.

If you take out the five hundred antibiotics, that still leaves 249,500 drugs—not a single one of which is designed to cure anything. Maybe antibiotics might cure strep throat or certain types of infections.

Other than that, there's not a single drug that actually cures anything. Drugs are all designed to milk your insurance policies. They're all designed to milk your wallet.

There is no law requiring the pharmaceutical companies to manufacture drugs that cure. Drugs don't cure. You cannot fix a nutritional deficiency with a drug.

It's No Laughing Matter

I've made thousands of tapes and gave presentations to audiences over the years, and I learned how to get laughs and nods of agreement and understanding from the audience. One of the toughest objections to deal with after a seminar or phone conference was, "That's all very interesting, Dr. Wallach, but I'm on two prescription medications, so I think I had better ask my doctor first."

Therefore, I decided I had to deal head on with the blind adoration and respect that the general public heaped upon doctors. I started the hobby of collecting articles on crimes that had been perpetrated by doctors. I even collected obituaries of young doctors to build a case against the medical profession's seemingly spotless image.

Statistics showing that a few doctors sexually abused their patients, that some actually murdered their spouses, patients, or partners, some were arsonists, and that some had embezzled money from Medicare brought laughs from the audience but didn't put a dent in the numbers of people who still wanted to "check with their doctor." Someone else's MD might be an ax murderer, but his or her personal doctor was still considered a medical god. But he or she is not. For many, the medical profession's credibility in the area of health knowledge had not been tarnished enough.

The End of Managed Healthcare

Health spending has surged. This is what American people asked for when they abolished managed care, and that is what they received.

For about 8 years, the cost of healthcare stayed the same when there was managed care. Doctors didn't like it, because managed care kept them from doing unnecessary tests. Managed healthcare kept them from doing unnecessary surgeries and writing prescriptions for unnecessary drugs. They didn't like it, because it cut their income in half. They weren't getting the kickbacks anymore.

So they began to whisper to their patients: There's a bookkeeper making decisions about what medications you should have, what tests you should have, and what treatments you should have. That should be my job, not a bookkeeper's job. I'm a doctor.

And after a while people said, yes, it should be the doctor's job. They asked, why is some bookkeeper doing the doctor's job?

So they convinced the American public that managed healthcare was bad. People complained to their legislators, and they voted out managed healthcare. Their workplaces went to things other than managed care.

Immediately, when managed healthcare got dumped, the spending for healthcare doubled, and tripled, and it's going up like a rocket because now there are no controls on the doctors.

How does this affect us? The age 65 and over workforce has risen sharply since 1980. People are worried about their financial security, and it's because of the cost of healthcare. As you get older, you need more healthcare.

Doctors are always going to get paid. You're going to pay them, your employer will pay them, or the government will pay them.

Someone's going to pay them. Doctors don't worry about where their next mortgage payment is coming from. They're confident they'll get paid.

THE REST OF US? WE WORRY ABOUT OUR PAYCHECKS.

One of the reasons we worry about our paychecks is because so many of our employers have outsourced so many U.S. jobs to other countries. That's partly because of healthcare spending.

In America, companies have to pay each full-time employee a salary plus healthcare benefits. If we outsource the jobs, we can pay employees a lower salary, and we don't have to include healthcare benefits in the compensation package.

As healthcare benefits climb, and companies don't want to pay for them anymore, these employers start outsourcing jobs to countries that don't have healthcare benefits.

What happens to the people who are here in the United States? They still have to pay for their healthcare somehow. They may not have the money to do it, but one way or another, the insurance companies will get their money. If individuals can't pay, then the taxes of other individuals will cover the insurance costs for them.

Meanwhile, doctors aren't missing a trip to the bank to deposit their paychecks. And they're not always very good at earning that money.

On the contrary, it's been widely reported that doctors skip key steps in treatments. They fail to take about half the recommended steps for treating common illnesses such as high blood pressure and diabetes, suggesting that healthcare in the United States isn't nearly as good as many people thought. That's not news.

Lying to Insurance Companies

Every so often, an unusually egregious case of a doctor who lies to insurance companies makes the news. Michigan-based Dr. Farid Fata was convicted of misdiagnosing patients with cancer—purposely!—and ordering treatment. As you know, chemotherapy, radiation, and other cancer treatments have side effects that can be deadly, and they can cost people their savings along with their health.

Dr. Fata was content to watch his patients' hair and teeth fall out just as long as he could pocket the money he received from their insurance companies for treatments they didn't need. He was also willing to treat terminally ill patients who couldn't benefit from cancer treatments in any way. In all, he victimized more than 500 patients. Of course, that was only one doctor, and he was sentenced to 45 years in jail.

His unfortunate patients, of course, have been sentenced to a lifetime of dealing with the side effects of trusting a physician who abused them to fatten his bank account.

In other news, USA Today reported in October 1999 that the problem of doctors committing insurance fraud is a lot more widespread than just one individual.

There was a study done in eight cities that looked at 169 internists and was presented to the American Medical Association's annual conference in Los Angeles. Fifty-eight percent of the internists supported lying to insurance companies so a severely ill 55-year-old could get a coronary bypass even though her pains were not increasing in frequency as the insurance company required during the managed care days.

Now, if your pains are not becoming more frequent, and the degree of pain remains the same, this is called stable angina. For a very modest monthly cost, you can put a nitroglycerin tablet under your tongue to deal with the pain. You can do that forever. Dean Ornish is a physician. He's the president and founder of the nonprofit Preventive Medicine Research Institute in Sausalito, California, and he's a Clinical Professor of Medicine at the University of California in San Francisco.

He did a great double-blind study where he took hundreds of people with 85% and 90% blockage of the three main coronary arteries, and he put them on a restricted diet. He gave them some supplements and some low-impact exercise like yoga and swimming. In six months, all of their arteries were open a hundred percent without surgery.

This was impossible, according to surgeons. The only way to deal with blocked arteries is to do a bypass, right? There's no way you can do that with diet, exercise, and supplements. So they made him repeat the study, and the results were exactly the same.

What a doctor should say today when someone comes to them with stable angina is, "Look, let's get you on restricted diet program. It will cut your food bill in half. We'll get you on a nutritional supplement program. Come back in six months, and if you've improved, then just keep doing the same thing. If it gets worse, then we'll consider the surgery." But there are no doctors who do that.

Doctors lie a little bit, but they want you to believe they're doing it for the good of their patients. Actually, the doctor isn't lying for the patient's benefit. The doctors lie for themselves, because they want the tens of thousands of dollars the surgeries would bring them. They want to keep that cash flow going.

A 1997 study by the Health Insurance Association of America found that seventy-five percent of insurance fraud is committed by providers. That's their code word for doctors. Doctors commit insurance fraud in two ways.

> **THEY APPLY FOR PAYMENT, WHICH THEY GET, FOR PROCEDURES THEY DIDN'T EVEN DO.**
>
> **THEY GET PAYMENT FOR PROCEDURES THEY GIVE YOU THAT YOU DIDN'T NEED.**

When doctors need money, they don't go to a bank like the rest of the professionals in this country. They just send in a couple of claims to an insurance company, and the insurance company pays them.

Every doctor should go to jail for that. Insurance companies simply write that off as a cost of doing business.

So who pays for that? We do. Each and every one of us pays for that as health insurance premiums go up, and as more and more doctors are doing these things. Doctors seem to look at it this way: "Hey, it's our money. We're entitled to it, and we're going to get it any way we can."

Carpenter With No Hammer Skills

In September of 1997, there was an article published in the Journal of the American Medical Association with the headline "Young Doctors Lack Stethoscope Skills." A stethoscope is one of the primary instruments of doctors. The report found that many doctors who had been steeped in high-tech medicine can't properly use a stethoscope.

With a stethoscope, they could identify only 20% of heart problems that were presented to them. They couldn't identify 80%. How can you go to medical school for fourteen years and not be able to use a stethoscope? That's like a carpenter apprenticing for seven years who doesn't know how to use a hammer.

The reason why doctors don't spend much time learning how to use a stethoscope is this. If they were to use a stethoscope to diagnose cardiovascular problems (and, by the way, you can identify all cardiovascular problems with a stethoscope), then they wouldn't have to send the patient off to get an angiogram, CT scan, MRI, or ultrasound. They'd make thirty dollars for an office visit instead of more than four-hundred dollars for sending someone in for one of those procedures.

Dead or Alive

Stories like this happen three thousand times a year in America. Eighty-six-year-old Mildred C. Clark was found cold, stiff, and blue on her apartment floor. The apartment manager got scared because he thought she was dead, so he called the paramedics. The paramedics came and examined her, and they couldn't find a heartbeat. So they called the coroner who came and agreed that she was dead. So they put her in a body bag and shipped her to the Albany, New York medical center, which is associated with a medical school in upstate New York. They sent an intern to do the final exam before they wrote a death certificate out for her, because you can't do an autopsy until somebody has a death certificate. So he examined her, and he probably just closed his eyes. He'd probably never seen a dead body by himself, so he wasn't checking too closely. So they took her down to the morgue, and they stripped her naked, and they took a pressure hose and cleaned her. Then they put her, wet, into the body bag and put her in the freezer for ninety minutes until the pathologist or medical examiner got there to do the autopsy.

Ninety minutes after putting her in the freezer, they wheeled her out and then noticed that the body bag was moving, and so they unzipped it, and eighty-six-year-old Mildred C. Clark sat up. She said, "Thank goodness you found me. It was cold and dark in there, and I didn't know where I was."

After fourteen years of medical school, doctors can't even tell if you're alive or dead. That makes me nervous.

Who Do You Trust?

Here are a few more things to make us all nervous. Each year:

- Doctors kill 300,000 patients in hospitals alone as a result of medical negligence.
- 1.3 million Americans are injured in hospitals as a result of medical negligence
- 2 million Americans are infected in hospitals. And, despite heroic around-the-clock nursing and antibiotics, 90,000 to 100,000 of these 2 million patients die.

- 2.2 million Americans get adverse drug reactions to the drugs they're introduced to in the hospital, and despite heroic measures, 140,000 to 200,000 die very year.

If you add up these numbers, that's between 3.5 million and 4 million casualties who are killed, injured, and infected each year in hospitals by doctors. The number is estimated to be double that outside of hospitals.

Now we're not talking about a few people a year. We're talking about a huge number of people. So why do we go to doctors for health and longevity information?

In 1999, doctors were believed to be the eighth top killer of Americans. Medical mistakes, specifically, were the eighth top killer of Americans, just behind cardiovascular disease, cancer, diabetes, Alzheimer's disease, gastro-intestinal problems, liver problems, and kidney problems.

Over the years, the numbers have shifted. Doctors are now listed as the number one cause of death in America. Number two is cardiovascular disease, and number three is cancer. It's a miracle if you survive a hospital visit without being damaged, infected, or killed.

Thomas Jefferson said that a little revolution once in a while is a good thing. It's time to revolt against the American healthcare system. Doctors do everything in their favor and nothing in their patients' favor.

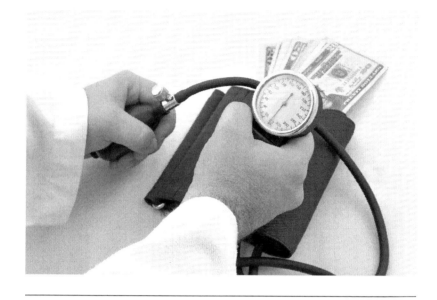

Talk About a Revolution

So how do we deal with this? We've learned, in other instances, how to handle it when the industry is abusing us. For example, sixty years ago, the automobile industry began to abuse customers. You'd go in for a six-dollar oil change, and you'd go to pick up your car, and they'd demand three hundred dollars. That was your month's wages. You'd say, what do you mean you want me to pay three-hundred dollars. The dealer would say, well, you told us to do whatever was necessary, so we rebuilt your transmission and your carburetor, and we gave you all new tires and rotated them, we put in new brake shoes and spark plugs, so that adds up to three hundred dollars. And you kicked the counter and yelled and screamed, but in the end, you paid your three hundred bucks. Well, people got tired of that so they started going to flea markets, junkyards, and garage sales looking for parts for the car. And, after a while, the demand for these parts and tools became so great that the flea markets, junkyards, and garage sales couldn't handle it anymore, so a whole new industry popped up. Chain stores that provided discounted parts like AutoZone and NAPA appeared. Now you can walk in and get any part you want. You can get any tool you need to work on your own car. This has turned out to be a huge industry.

> **BECAUSE THE AUTOMOBILE INDUSTRY GOT GREEDY SIXTY YEARS AGO, MORE PEOPLE FIX THEIR OWN CARS NOW.**

The same thing happened in the construction industry. It got to the point where they were charging people sixty dollars to change a float in the toilet or two hundred dollars to change a light bulb. Or you'd sign a contract to pay six thousand dollars for a new roof, but they didn't tell you about the revolving interest factor, and if you didn't pay it in the year, it would cost you a hundred thousand dollars. As all these horror stories came to light, people began shopping at flea markets, junkyards, and garage sales looking for materials to repair their own homes. So, since the supply couldn't keep up with the demand, new stores came on board, and they were called The Home Depot, Lowe's, and others. If you don't know how to put shingles on your own roof or tile your own floor, they'll give you a free class.

Well, it's long overdue that we rebel against the healthcare industry. You can do more yourself. With a little bit of education, 15 minutes of reading per night, listening to CDs or mp3s as you drive in your car, you can be your own doctor when it comes to giving yourself advice and helping yourself live healthier, longer.

IT'S THAT SIMPLE.

For example, a doctor has a hundred-dollars' worth of stuff in his examining room. He has a blood pressure cuff, a stethoscope, a thermometer, a little rubber mallet to check your reflexes, a little, triple-A battery penlight to look in your eyes and down your throat (and that was given to the doctor by a salesperson from a pharmaceutical company). You can go to a pharmacy or a big box store and buy all those supplies for yourself without a prescription. With the exception of ultrasound, radiation, MRIs, and CT scans, you can get just about any test that a doctor would send you to a lab or a hospital to get.

For instance, you can buy a little bottle of test strips to find out what your blood sugar and blood cholesterol is. You can get test strips to find out if you have sugar or blood in your urine. You can get test strips to find out if you have blood in your bowel movement, and do a screen for colon cancer, and also colitis and gastric ulcers.

You can do a home pregnancy test. You don't have to get a medical exam, and then come back in three days for another medical exam that doubles the price, just to find out if you're pregnant or not.

Fertility clinics are even more difficult to justify. You have to pay thousands of dollars up front before they even talk to you, because they're afraid they might slip and give you some information that you can use on your own. So, before the doctor will see you, you have to pay the fee. Then, once you've paid that, they'll start talking to you about what they can do to help you in a situation of infertility. They want you to believe that they are the keepers of all the knowledge about this. Back when I was a kid, my dad only had a fourth grade education, and he knew how to artificially inseminate cattle. This isn't a new thing. We've been doing it with livestock for nearly a century. Any farmer can do artificial insemination.

With a couple of items that cost less than five dollars, you can do it yourself. And we're paying fertility clinics tens of thousands of dollars!

So when a doctor starts telling you how technical these things are, they are hoping you will blindly smile and say ok.

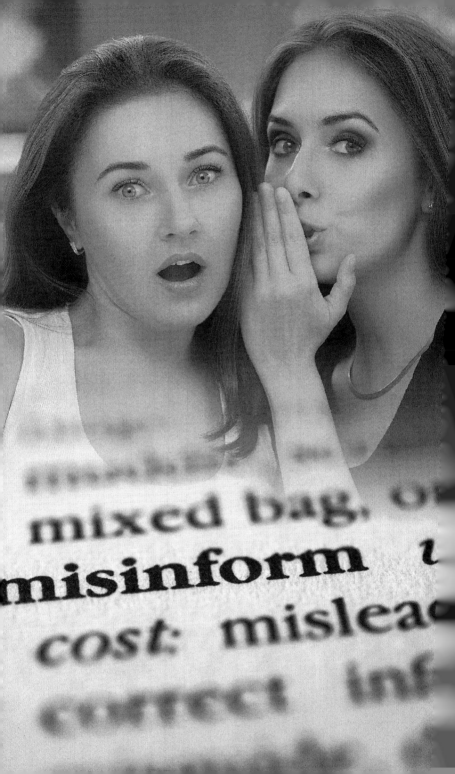

CHAPTER 6

MISINFORMATION ABOUNDS

The Yolk's on Us

Each year in America, we spend over a hundred billion dollars for cholesterol testing—not treatment, but testing. It's a huge industry. That's why doctors have made us all paranoid about cholesterol.

If you've had someone in your family live to be in their eighties or nineties, and most people have, I guarantee you they ate eggs instead of Eggbeaters, they cooked in butter because they didn't have margarine back then, they salted their food, they could have smoked, they ate red meat instead of tofu, and they didn't have gym memberships. Yet they lived long, healthy lives. Following the advice of modern-day doctors, we're going backward. We're spending a hundred billion dollars a year for cholesterol-level testing, and we're eating the way doctors have told us, because most people revere their doctors. And we've gone from 17th in the world for longevity to 40th. So it doesn't seem as if all of that is doing much good.

No one has ever found a disease that's caused by elevated cholesterol and triglycerides. When you have elevated cholesterol and triglycerides, I look for other things. You might have a deficiency of niacin, vitamin B3. You might have a deficiency of chromium and vanadium, two trace minerals. You might have deficiencies of fatty acids, or a ratio problem between omega 3 and omega 6. You might have early goiter or hypothyroidism. You might have early diabetes. Even before your blood sugar goes up, your blood cholesterol and triglycerides go up.

Don't take my word for it. Go to the library, and look in a medical book of diagnoses. You'll see the first blood changes that occur when you have diabetes. Your blood cholesterol and triglycerides go up. You'll see the first blood changes that occur when you have hypothyroidism. Your blood cholesterol and triglycerides go up again. Do the elevated blood cholesterol and triglycerides cause any disease? No. They're just signals to look somewhere. Do they cause cardiovascular disease? No. They have nothing to do with cardiovascular disease. Nothing.

Why do doctors get so excited about lowering your cholesterol and lowering your blood triglycerides? Because they get a kickback every time they write a prescription for statin drugs: Lipitor, Levacor, Zocor, Pravachol, Crestor, and the like.

Why would you take a drug that doesn't really do anything to prevent diseases, but instead causes liver cirrhosis and blindness and other horrible real diseases? That's why you have to go to the doctor every couple of months. They have to take a look and see how your liver is doing and look at your eye to make sure you're not going blind yet. It's a win-win for the doctors who can get a healthy person to take a harmful drug for no reason. They trick you into taking a statin drug, which you didn't need in the first place. And now you end up with real problems because of the drug and you go back to the same doctor who in essence gave you the diseases in the first place. And then they pile on more drugs and the cycle continues.

It's like going to a mechanic with a brand new car, and they end up tricking you into subjecting the car to expensive unnecessary tests and then putting water in the gas tank so that you can come back later with real issues.

Free radicals. Trans-fatty acids. These are common words today. Even six-year olds know about these things. These are the bad foods, and yet doctors continue to recommend that we consume them. I can prove it.

But first, let me ask you this. If I were to come out with a product, Dr. Wallach's 100 Percent Pure Free Radicals, the finest trans-fatty acids in the world, and I labeled them and put them in a health food store, how many people would buy them? Zero. I wouldn't sell any of them.

And yet everyone listens to doctors when they say, "I want you to use margarine instead of butter." Margarine is nothing but a big block of trans-fatty acids and free radicals. It is pure, 100% trans-fatty acids and free radicals. And it is the worst kind of fat for hearts. They've killed more people in America with margarine than all the wars—both domestic and foreign—put together in the two hundred plus years this country has been in existence.

If you have any margarine at home now, I'd like you to box it all up and ship it out to terrorists. Put a little note in there that says, "My cardiologist says this is good for your heart. So, as a show of good faith, I'm sending you some." Hopefully, they'll be stupid enough to use it. I like to have my patients eat between six and eight eggs a day. The more eggs you eat, the better. They're a great protein. They have a lot of good stuff in them, and I recommend soft scrambling them in butter or soft poaching them or cooking them over easy.

In 1995, when a study was published saying that two eggs a day were harmless, it sent shock waves throughout our medical system. At that time, eggs were the father of the devil. If you ate eggs, you were doomed. Nobody would hang around you. They'd say, "He's an egg eater" and make the sign of the cross to ward you off.

In March of 1991, the New England Journal of Medicine published a story about an 88-year-old man who ate 25 eggs each day and had normal plasma cholesterol. You have to ask yourself why this man was eating 25 eggs a day. Maybe he didn't have any teeth and couldn't eat steaks anymore. Maybe he owned an egg farm and liked to do his own quality control. But I think it was more scientific than that.

Ninety-five percent of the male sex hormone, testosterone, and ninety-five percent of the female sex hormones, estrogen and progesterone, 95% of the weight of our adrenal hormones, adrenaline, comes from a master steroid in our body called cholesterol. We only make ten percent. The other ninety percent must come from our diet.

When your adrenal glands are exhausted, what's the most likely thing that you're not consuming enough of? Cholesterol.

When your wife has you on a butter-free, egg-free, red meat-free diet, and you're more interested in watching the television than in watching her wear her new nightgown and enjoying a romantic evening together, maybe you're just not eating enough cholesterol.

Could Alzheimer's Disease Be Doctor Inflicted?

Alzheimer's disease is a physician-caused disease. This disease did not occur, even by another name, going back half a century. It became recognized as a disease in 1979. It became the number-five killer of adults over the age of 65 behind doctors, cardiovascular disease, cancer, and diabetes.

Myelin is a fatty insulation material that makes up 75% of our brain weight. It's so important to the human and animal brain.

And myelin is one hundred percent cholesterol. Remember, you can only make ten percent of your daily need for cholesterol. The other ninety percent must come from your food.

So if you're very good at following your doctor's advice, and you give up eating eggs and eat only Eggbeaters, if you give up butter and you eat margarine, if you give up eating red meat and eat only tofu, if you rip the chicken skin off the chicken before you eat it, and especially if you are taking a cholesterol restricting drug, the odds are that you're going to get Alzheimer's disease.

As baby boomers age, they're especially at risk of getting Alzheimer's disease, because they listen to their doctors. They believe in technology. They believe that, if they follow their doctors' advice, they can live to be 100. So a higher percentage of baby boomers get Alzheimer's disease than our grandparents did. Our grandparents, remember, ate everything they could afford to eat including red meat, eggs, and butter when it was available for them.

We eliminated Alzheimer's disease in animals more than 65 years ago.

This is a human study that came out in July of 1992. The University of California at San Diego Medical School and the Salk Institute found that vitamin E can ease memory loss in Alzheimer's patients and help them function again. Of course, no one could believe that was true, so they did the study again. Five years later, the UCSD Medical School released the results: high doses of common vitamin E might slow Alzheimer's disease for some patients which would significantly delay the need for nursing home care.

It would be emotionally and financially beneficial to children, grandchildren, nieces, and nephews if they could postpone the need for nursing care for their loved ones, right? But doctors don't tell them about the potential benefits of vitamin E because they own the stock in the nursing homes. They don't want this information to get out.

In November of 2003, a study by Tufts University Medical School found that you could reduce your risk of Alzheimer's disease by 48% by taking supplements or eating fish three times a day to get the omega-3 essential fatty acids. This study has been repeated over and over.

In January of 2004, people taking vitamin C and E were 78% less likely to have a diagnosis of Alzheimer's disease. They didn't even think about the diet, or try to get rid of fried foods, margarine, or other sources of free radicals. They didn't even think about eating cholesterol. They just ingested some antioxidants. So we know from animal studies and these early studies in human beings that if you eat enough cholesterol—eggs that are not fried, and not cooked in margarine, but poached, boiled, or scrambled in butter, and meat medium rare—and take in antioxidants, the odds of your getting Alzheimer's disease are reduced to almost zero.

This Raises My Blood Pressure

Blood pressure is a common disease. Have you ever heard of a veterinarian recommending that you give your dog a calcium channel blocker or a beta blocker for high blood pressure? What about your goldfish? What about your parakeet and guinea pig?

Every animal can get high blood pressure just as people do. The reason they don't is that in their little pellets of food that we've formulated for their needs, we've added things so they don't get high blood pressure.

WHEN WAS THE LAST TIME YOU SAW A GOLDFISH TAKING A HIGH BLOOD PRESSURE PILL?

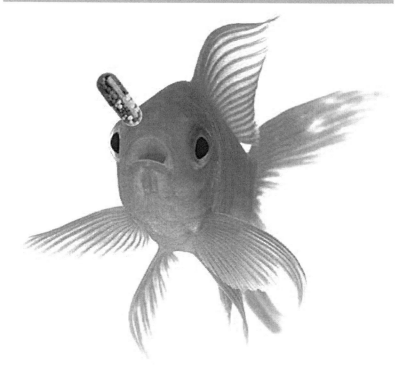

They can get high blood pressure. But they don't get it, because we put things in their food to ensure they don't get it.

You've heard that salt can cause high blood pressure. You've heard that genetics has something to do with causing high blood pressure, too.

Both of those myths are false. Salt and genetics have nothing to do with high blood pressure.

High blood pressure is the simple deficiency of a simple nutrient. It's one simple mineral.

> **HIGH BLOOD PRESSURE COMES DOWN TO THIS. YOU'RE MISSING A SINGLE MINERAL.**

We've eliminated high blood pressure in all of our animals. What's the first thing a good farmer puts down for his livestock in the pasture? A salt block or a salt lick, and there's no one out in the pasture telling a cow or a sheep that she's limited to one lick each day.

I refuse to believe that my human patients are stupider than a cow or a sheep. So I tell them to salt their food to taste, and don't worry about it.

Remember the Japanese. They consume an entire salt shaker per person in a day—that's 15 grams of salt. And they have 85% less cardiovascular disease than we do, and high blood pressure isn't even in their vocabulary because they don't get it very often.

In July of 1997, it was reported that researchers have no proof that too much salt is unhealthful even though doctors had been advising their patients to cut back on their salt intake for years. When doctors give bad advice for money, we call them quacks.

So next time your doctor tells you that you have to cut back on your salt intake because of your age, you can call your doctor a quack.

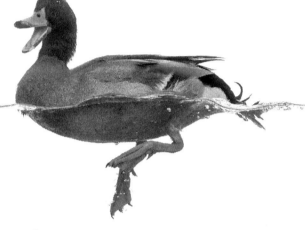

You can say, "You have no evidence to support that recommendation. I know you want to give me a prescription for statin drugs and blood pressure medication even though I don't have those problems, but you need to go back and read your stuff here. Because you have misinformation."

There was a wonderful study done by the U.S. government called the Sodium Task Force. They were trying to prove, once and for all, that salt was the cause of high blood pressure. This was published in April of 1997.

The study found that people who limited their salt intake to 1,000 milligrams a day as doctors recommend have six times more heart attacks than those who consume more than 2,400 milligrams of salt a day.

If you listened to your doctor, you had six times the number of heart attacks than people who defied their doctors and ate double the amount of salt they were told was their upper limit. So what are we really talking about when it comes to high blood pressure? It turns out that high blood pressure is a deficiency of a single mineral: calcium.

You can drink fifty gallons of milk a day, and you can't get enough calcium to get your high blood pressure down.

You can eat twenty-five pounds of cheese a day, and you still won't get enough calcium to lower your high blood pressure. The only thing you'll get is constipated.

You can take all the Tums you want. You can take all the oyster shells, egg shells, limestone, or oral calcium that you want. It won't affect your blood pressure. That's because if you take calcium carbonate, which is the chemical compound name for all of those substances, it is difficult for your body to digest and absorb. You will only be getting ten percent of the calcium you think you're getting. That isn't enough. I take a calcium supplement that is almost 100% absorbable. I also take the rest of the other 90 essential nutrients in an absorbable and usable form. Hopefully you are, too.

What Price Menopause?

Up until 1958, every doctor used to make a bit of pocket change dispensing an herbal formula called Lydia Pinkham which was named after Lydia Estes Pinkham, the inventor of the herbal tonic that relieved a woman's menstrual cramps and got rid of the hot flashes and night sweats. But doctors only made fifty cents when they dispensed a bottle.

In 1958, the pharmaceutical companies came out with HRT, Hormone Replacement Therapy. All the research was done by veterinarians, and they were told not to give it to humans because it did terrible things to the laboratory animals. But, because lab animals aren't humans, they wanted to see what would happen to women who used it, and they began to give it to them in 1958. Doctors would make a lot more money recommending HRT, so that is what they did.

It turns out that HRT, estrogen and progesterone combinations, increase the risk of breast, uterine, and ovarian cancer by 78%. It increases the risk of dementia and Alzheimer's disease by 200%. It increases the risk of cardiovascular disease by 200%. It increases your risk of asthma by 100%. It increases your risk of gradual deafness as you get older by 30%.

WHY WOULD ANYBODY WANT TO TAKE HRT?

You want to get rid of the hot flashes and night sweats any way you can. But why would you risk all these terrible things?

Women's thoughts, as a man, I just didn't understand. I went back and put together a formula similar to the original Lydia Pinkham formula, and guess what? It works like a charm. I even added a bunch of minerals to the herbal recipe. I call it Women's Fx.

There are dozens of major studies that show those herbs get rid of the hot flashes and night sweats. Then you throw in the liquid calcium, 1,200 milligrams per serving, and you deal with the concerns about osteoporosis, too.

And you don't have to deal with the risks from the HRT.

> **WOMEN'S FX FORMULA PLUS LIQUID CALCIUM EQUALS THE END OF HOT FLASHES AND NIGHT SWEATS.**

But Weight There's More!

Forty percent of Americans are overweight now. They weigh at least thirty pounds more than the ideal weight for their body type, height, and so forth.

This is a relatively new problem. Half a century ago, about fifteen percent of Americans were obese. A century ago, you very rarely saw an obese person in America. Less than one percent of all Americans were obese then.

> **OBESITY IS CAUSED BY A SIMPLE PROBLEM.**

When I walk around a horse farm, I can tell you in just a few minutes whether the horses are getting all the minerals they need. When horses lick the farmer's hot, sweaty hands, they are licking the salt.

My dad, with his fourth-grade education, knew that every time he'd see our cattle chewing on the fence and eating dirt, and chewing on the feedbox instead of eating the feed, that they were mineral deficient. He'd give them minerals, and they'd get back to their normal eating habits. The abhorrent eating behaviors would go away.

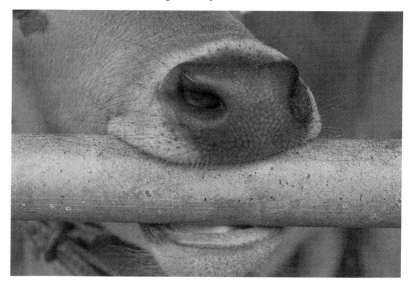

We usually learn in our childhoods that it is not socially acceptable to chew on the furniture and eat dirt. "If you're that hungry, go into the kitchen and have a piece of pie with ice cream," your parents tell you. "Or have a Twinkie."

People began to recognize these cravings, which we call pica disorder in animals and the munchies in people. We've been taught that these cravings are due to a Twinkie deficiency. If we were taught, as kids, that this was caused by a mineral deficiency, we'd all take minerals that have zero calories in them. Americans would all be slim.

Weight problems are nothing more than a mineral deficiency disorder. No one knows more about weight gain and weight loss than veterinarians. When you put an animal into the feed lot, what are they supposed to do? Lose weight or gain weight? Gain weight, obviously. We know the technology, and so do snack food companies. They spend a lot of money on research learning the technology of weight gain. They manufacture their snacks to make sure it's hard to eat just one of them or one of those unsatisfying little 100-calorie packages. LAY'S® potato chips is even using that as their motto. Bet you can't eat just one!

They fix it so that you're mineral deficient if you eat their snack foods. But, if you take your minerals, the cravings go away. That alone will reduce snacking. You'll lose ten, fifteen, or twenty pounds because you're not craving food between meals. You won't sit in front of the television set and stuff yourself with snacks all night, because you won't have those cravings anymore.

- It's not a problem with your willpower or your self-respect.
- You don't have a deficiency of hypnosis or acupuncture.
- You don't have a deficiency of a weight loss drug.
- You have deficiencies of minerals.

You take your minerals, and you take a couple of meal replacers each day. You give up some carbohydrates in your breads, pastas, rice, and potatoes. And you're going to lose weight and keep it off. The weight won't come back as long as you stay on that program. As soon as you go off your minerals, the cravings start up again, because you'll have a mineral deficiency.
You can get rid of the mineral deficiencies rather easy. You need the 90 essential nutrients and you need them in a form that is easily absorbable

CHAPTER 7

THREE SERIOUS TOPICS

Cancer, War, and Lies

Now I want to talk about a serious topic: cancer. In 1997, an article was published in USA Today with the headline 30 Billion Dollar War on Cancer a Bust? A bill was signed by President Nixon when he was in office to spend 30 billion dollars on the war against cancer. Despite spending the money, researchers suggest putting emphasis on preventing cancer instead of curing it.

IF YOU WERE A MEDICAL RESEARCHER, WHAT COULD YOU DO WITH 30 BILLION DOLLARS?

If you give me 30 billion dollars, in one year, I'll find a cure. For 30 billion dollars, why couldn't researchers find a cure for cancer? It only took 100-million dollars to fly an astronaut to the moon, put him on the surface of the moon, and bring him back home again.

Researchers could absolutely have found a cancer cure for 30-billion dollars, but they didn't think outside the box. They weren't really looking for a cure. They spent all their time looking for better chemotherapy with your tax money, because that's where the money is. During that time, every five years, they doubled the amount of money they used for research. The death toll remained the same. So they obviously weren't looking in the right place, and they couldn't have been looking that hard.

In October of 1998, a Harvard Nurses' Health Study was published that found multivitamins cut colon cancer. The study had 90,000 nurses and 20 years of data. They could only use 15 years of the 20 years of data in this study because, for the first 5 years, there weren't enough nurses using multivitamins.

The study concluded that the 90,000 nurses who were taking multivitamins for at least 15 years cut their risk of colon cancer by 75%. There are no drugs on the market that will do that. Why didn't your doctors email or call you and let you know that, just by taking one multivitamin a day, you could reduce your risk of colon cancer by 75%? They read about it in their medical journals, but that is not good news for their business, so they will pretend not to know. They may even make themselves not believe it.

The common wisdom is that low-fat diets, too, will reduce your risk of colon cancer and breast cancer. High-fat diets, the doctors tell you, increase your risk of cancer.

However, in March of 1999, the Journal of the American Medical Association published an article with the headline, "No link between fat, breast cancer."

In a study of 90,000 nurses, they compared the rate of cancer of those who had more than fifty percent of their calories as fat (which is a very high fat diet) to those who had less than twenty percent of their calories as fat (which is a very low fat diet).

If the fat content of your diet had anything to do with the rate of cancer, then the nurses having more than fifty percent of their calories as fat should have a lot more cancer than the people having less than twenty percent of their calories as fat.

However, the study found no measurable difference between the cancer rates of the two groups. Contrary to what you've always heard, the amount of fat in your diet has nothing to do with the rate of cancer. What matters isn't the amount of fat that you have in your diet. It's how you cook the fat that counts.

In 1998, a big University of South Carolina study linked well-done meat to breast cancer and, later on, to prostate cancer and colon cancer. Among women who preferred all of their meat to be cooked very well-done, there was a 462% greater chance of having breast cancer than for women who ate their meat rare or medium.

ASKING FOR YOUR BURGERS AND STEAKS TO BE COOKED WELL DONE IS JUST LIKE ASKING FOR CANCER.

Burned animal fat, whether it's in hot dog skins or grilled chicken skin or hamburgers, will increase your risk of breast cancer, prostate cancer, and colon cancer by 462%. Now that you know, it's easy to make the decision to change your habit of eating burned animal fat.

The wisdom also says that a high-fiber diet reduces your risk of colon cancer. That's another one of those truisms that your doctor and the American Cancer Society want you to believe. Quaker Oats likes that myth, too, because it helps them sell a lot of oatmeal.

MYTH: A HIGH-FIBER DIET LOWERS YOUR RISK OF COLON CANCER.

The New England Journal of Medicine published a Harvard Nurses' Health Study of 90,000 nurses in January of 1999. Researchers compared the rate of colon cancer of those who had a high-fiber diet with those who had a low-fiber diet.

They didn't like the results, so they threw in 50,000 male doctors. They compared the rate of colon cancers, too, of those doctors who had a high-fiber diet with those who had a low-fiber diet. Now they had 140,000 human subjects.

Their finding was that high-fiber diets do not cut the rate of colon cancer by any measurable amount. Eating a high-fiber diet did not protect you in any way, shape, or form from getting colon cancer.

Why do doctors get so excited about a high-fiber diet? It will reduce your cholesterol.

It does that because it absorbs everything you eat including minerals that are required to keep you from getting high blood pressure, osteoporosis, arthritis, and cancer.

So people who eat multi-grain breads for their toast, English muffins, waffles, and pancakes for breakfast, and people who eat multi-grain pastas, actually have a five hundred percent greater risk of all these degenerative diseases that kill you.

That means that, by eating a high-fiber diet, your risk of all those other diseases goes up. At the same time, your risk of colon cancer does not decrease at all. The only thing the doctors get excited about regarding eating a high-fiber diet is that it lowers your cholesterol. And does that do anything positive for you?

No. It doesn't do a single positive thing.

THIS IS BERRY GOOD NEWS.

According to an Ohio University study, you reduce your risk of colon cancer by sixty to eighty percent by eating dark berries: raspberries, blueberries, blackberries, black raspberries, black cherries, and strawberries.

Have you heard that a trace mineral, selenium, is a great antioxidant that can reduce your risk of cancer? That sounds pretty exciting, doesn't it?

SELENIUM CAN SLASH THE OCCURRENCE OF PROSTATE CANCER BY 69 PERCENT.

In fact, the information about selenium really came out in April of 1912 and was published in Popular Mechanics Magazine. A professor from Berlin, Dr. August von Wasserman, who went on about ten years later to win a Nobel Prize in medicine, said that he had discovered a chemical substance that would cure cancer in mice. It turns out that chemical substance was the trace mineral selenium. He said that selenium had a selective action against cancer cells that doesn't hurt healthy tissues.

Dr. Wasserman believed the cancers in mice were so similar to those in humans that he believed a significant advance had been made in learning how to cure cancers in people.

We began to put selenium into food pellets for animals to keep their rate of cancer down. Veterinarians have been using selenium for animals ever since. However, this lay dormant for 84 years in human medicine and nutrition until December of 1996. A seven-year study came out that was done by Dr. Larry Clark, an MD, Ph.D, from the University of Arizona School of Medicine. He took half a group of 1,300 people and gave them 200 micrograms of selenium every day for seven years.

At the end of the study, his final analysis showed that he slashed the occurrence—not the risk, but the occurrence—of prostate cancer by sixty-nine percent. Are there any drugs that can do that? Will doing a prostate exam and taking your PSA blood test every year prevent prostate cancer by sixty-nine percent? No. He reduced the occurrence of colorectal cancer by 64%. He reduced it by 75% by adding a multivitamin. He reduced the occurrence of lung cancer by 39% whether his subjects smoked or not.

Two months after this study came out, Dr. Larry Clark died of prostate cancer at age 52. Why did that happen? His study showed that selenium worked, but he set it up hoping to discredit selenium. He hated selenium. He wouldn't take it.

The worst part of all is that he was a professor of medicine at the Medical School of the University of Arizona. So he taught his beliefs to all the medical students there.

When he died of prostate cancer, they all said, "Oh, what a tragedy." Then they went on to become doctors who avoided selenium and who told their patients not to take selenium. Doctors choose which studies to believe. They like the studies that help them make more money. Doctors don't make much selling selenium. I'd be glad if they did. March 6, 2002, a study said that a diet rich in raw tomatoes can cut the risk of prostate cancer by 24 to 36%. If you eat tomatoes cooked, one serving a day will cut the risk of prostate cancer by 52 to 60% because there's an antioxidant in tomatoes called lycopene.

GREEN TEA IS A CURE-ALL OF CURE-ALLS.

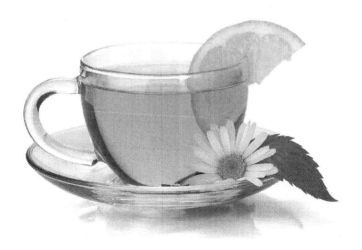

In September of 1998, a study came out that called green tea a cure-all of cure-alls. Why is that important? Why do we have 85% more cancer than the Japanese?

Our national drink is Coca-Cola. Their national drink is green tea, and green tea contains antioxidants called catechins (EGCG) that are a hundred times more potent than vitamin C in neutralizing free radicals and perhaps a hundred times more effective than vitamin C in reducing your risk of cancer.

The Diabetes Epidemic: Who's to Blame?

Diabetes is an epidemic disease in the United States. There are more than a million new cases diagnosed every year. In 2012, there were 29.1 million American diabetics. Of those, only 21 million had been diagnosed. That left 8.1 million Americans with undiagnosed cases of diabetes.

In older Americans, age 65 and up, 25.9% or 11.8 million seniors, had diabetes (both diagnosed an undiagnosed). Adult-onset diabetics make more insulin than non-diabetics. There isn't an insulin problem with them. So if you have insulin, how can you be a diabetic? The doctor will tell you that you have insulin-resistant diabetes. The insulin isn't working for you.

IF YOU HAVE INSULIN-RESISTANT DIABETES, YOU'RE MISSING THE TRACE MINERALS CHROMIUM/VANADIUM.

The reason it isn't working is that you're deficient in two trace minerals: chromium and vanadium. You can make tons of insulin, but if you don't have those two trace minerals, your insulin isn't going to work.

We learned in 1957 that we could prevent and cure adult-onset type diabetes in laboratory animals, pet animals, and farm animals by giving them these two trace minerals and their cofactors. This lay dormant for 20 years in human medicine until 1977.

At that time, they found out that they could give intravenous chromium/vanadium and their cofactors to people who had diabetes and were unconscious from head injuries. They were in a coma, and giving them these trace minerals and their cofactors miraculously cured them. You can't credit the placebo effect and say they were cured because they thought they would get cured. They were in a coma! They didn't know what was going on.

> **IT WAS THE TRACE MINERALS, CHROMIUM/VANADIUM, AND THEIR COFACTORS THAT CURED THE DIABETIC PEOPLE.**

Why doesn't your doctor tell you these things? The news has been published in every major medical journal. If the doctor took the time to share this information with you, he might get eighty dollars for an extended visit instead of fifty dollars for a standard visit. He'll make an extra thirty dollars. According to the General Accounting Office (GAO), which is the budget watchdog for the U.S. Congress, in the 25 to 40 years a diabetic lives after diagnosis, your doctor makes $750,000.

Why would he take thirty dollars when he can make $750,000?

Most people think, "but my doctor belongs to my church." Well, your doctor's religious practices won't protect you. Even members of the Mafia go to church, right? So don't assume that you can trust your doctor just because he's a religious man. He cares far more about his income than he does about you. It's not even a close call.

Marcus Welby, MD was just a fictional character. He never existed in the real world.

According to the U.S. Department of Agriculture, a hundred years ago, Americans were eating half a pound of sugar per person each year. A hundred years later, American are eating 157 pounds of sugar. That means we're eating half a pound of sugar each day. Combined with a deficiency of nutrients in our food, eating way too much sugar and not getting the best information available from our doctors has resulted in this epidemic of diabetes.

Do you think our genetics have changed that much? I don't think so.

Since the mid-1940s, the chromium levels in our blood have plummeting like a rock almost every year. In the late seventies, people were reading about the benefits of chromium and vanadium, and they were rushing to their health food stores and asking for it. So, for a couple of years, the levels of chromium in our blood went up.

But you can't cure diabetes with only chromium and vanadium

without its cofactors. So the levels of chromium in our blood decreased again, because people got frustrated and stopped taking it.

So between not having enough of these nutrients, the chromium and vanadium and its cofactors in our food anymore, and eating all this sugar, we have an epidemic of adult-onset type diabetes.

Who's to blame for the diabetes epidemic? In effect, we are, because we've been making really bad choices.

Make No Bones About It

According to the Center for Disease Control, eighty-five percent of all Americans over the age of fifty already have arthritis and osteoporosis of one type or another. There's not a single medical treatment designed to prevent or cure it.

Aspirin, Celebrex, Tylenol, Ibuprofen, Advil, Aleve, Methotrexate, Prednisone, or others. They all have side effects that can be life threatening.

As I write this, the U.S. Food and Drug Administration has reviewed new safety information, and because of that, it is calling upon the makers of some of these painkillers to strengthen the warnings on their labels. Taking NSAIDs, which are non-aspirin, nonsteroidal, anti-inflammatory drugs, creates an increased risk of a heart attack or a stroke.

The FDA is taking this new information seriously, and so should each one of us.

Painkillers aren't the way to deal with arthritis and osteoporosis. And what makes this especially ugly is that we've known that for hundreds of years.

> **WE DO KNOW HOW TO PREVENT AND CURE ARTHRITIS AND OSTEOPOROSIS, AND IT'S NOT THROUGH PAINKILLERS.**

We learned how to prevent and cure arthritis and osteoporosis in animals more than three hundred years ago. We didn't know all the chemical reasons why these approaches worked. But, for the last 75 years, we've known the biochemical reasons why these nutritional formulas worked.

So, yes, we've been preventing and curing arthritis and osteoporosis in animals for hundreds of years. Preventing and curing arthritis and osteoporosis is already a done deal.

And your doctors are still trying to give you painkillers, and they're doing surgery.

> **HOW MUCH IS ARTHROSCOPIC SURGERY OF THE KNEE WORTH? TO YOU, NOT A THING. TO DOCTORS, MILLIONS OF DOLLARS.**

You've heard of arthroscopic surgery of the knee for arthritis. It's a very common procedure now. In July 2002, there was a report published in The New England Journal of Medicine that called arthroscopic surgery for arthritis a worthless procedure.

If you have arthroscopic surgery, that doesn't deal with the systemic problem that's going on, you just have the promise of preserving your knee for a year or two and delaying joint-replacement surgery. There are only 5,000 doctors out of the one million doctors who do this procedure. In 2001, their income for doing just this one procedure was $1.5 billion. Given that, do you think they'll ever give up that procedure? No.

They're not going to use a nutritional approach that will actually work. They're going to use surgery, because that's more lucrative for them, even though it's completely worthless to patients.

If a doctor tries to sell you on arthroscopic surgery, and wants to take out those pieces of floating bone and cartilage, you have to be smart enough to say to the doctor: "You're a quack. How many people did you kill last month? The New England Journal of Medicine in July of 2002 said this procedure's worthless. Now, we've been friends a long time. And you're coming to me with a worthless procedure and recommending that I do it? I don't think I'm going to visit you anymore."

Otherwise, they'll keep taking advantage of you to milk your insurance policy and your wallet. You have to rebel sometime.

You might rebel when you realize your doctor is only looking at you as a source of income.

Maybe you've heard that osteoporosis is a post-menopausal woman's problem. Everyone "knows" that these days.

But we knew, more than a hundred years ago, that osteoporosis actually occurs equally in both men and women. It only became a post-menopausal woman's problem in 1958 when they came out with HRT, hormone replacement therapy.

Can you justify treating osteoporosis in women with estrogen when men and women get osteoporosis at the same rate? Just try to imagine a red-blooded American country man from Idaho going to his doctor and saying, "Okay. I have that osteoporosis disease. Give me some estrogen, please."

> **IT'S NOT GOING TO HAPPEN.
> PEOPLE ARE BASICALLY SMART.**

In November of 2001, the report came out from the Canadian Multicentre Osteoporosis Study that osteoporosis strikes both sexes equally. Men are as likely as women to suffer from osteoporosis. This was a surprise finding. All the doctors who did that study graduated after 1958, and the truth they were taught was that osteoporosis strikes only post-menopausal women.

The Canadian Multicentre Osteoporosis Study involved almost 10,000 participants in nine centers across Canada. It was predicted to change the way unexplained bone fractures in men were dealt with and the way education about the condition is handled.

Doctors don't share that information because they know, if they did, women immediately would stop using hormone replacement therapy to prevent osteoporosis.

And doctors are making so much money from the kickbacks as they write prescriptions for HRT that they're afraid to rock the boat. They don't want to start anything that's going to threaten that source of income.

So any doctor who continues today to write prescriptions for women for HRT should be put in jail for 25 years to life without the possibility of parole. That would be the kindest treatment I would recommend for them.

Ladies, when your doctor comes to you and says, "I want you to take estrogen for osteoporosis," you say, "Doctor, how about if you take it for 25 years? Then, if it works, I'll take it." See what he says.

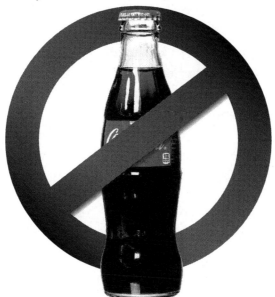

One of the other things you have to do besides taking all the raw materials to rebuild your bone, cartilage, ligaments, tendons, and connective tissue is to give up carbonated drinks. Carbonated drinks are the single greatest contributor to osteoporosis, arthritis, and fractures of the bone. They interfere with the absorption of nutrients, especially minerals, and digesting protein.

Pour the Soda Pop Down the Drain

The original study was done with the Harvard Nurses' Health Study. In 90,000 nurses over age 35, 20 years of data, they found out that the nurses drinking carbonated soft drinks—even diet drinks—instead of water during the day had a five hundred percent increase in their risk of osteoporosis and fractures over the water-drinking group.

Later, there was a Harvard study involving 460 girls in ninth and tenth grade that found the teenagers who drank carbonated beverages, especially cola, were more likely to break their bones.

Why did the studies only look at nurses and girls? Because the researchers believed osteoporosis was primarily a female disease.

But, believe me, it occurs in males, too. So if you have teenage athletes of either gender, and if you have osteoporosis or arthritis in your family—or if you either have it, or don't want to get it—you have to give up carbonated drinks.

Doctors should be telling you this every time you walk in the door. "You have to give up carbonated drinks." They do not.

Most of them drink it themselves. They also live shorter lives than the rest of us, too.

I just want to remind you that if you don't take care of your own destiny—if you don't take hold of things—life is going to take care of your destiny for you. And it probably won't be a very nice destiny.

So take control and rebel a little bit. Become one of those feisty people who defy their doctor.

But do it with education. You can't just break the rules without knowing what you're doing and why you're doing it.

> **EDUCATION IS POWER. EDUCATION WITH ACTION IS SUPERPOWER.**

In Conclusion

Standard, orthodox medical doctors used to tell their patients that diet and supplements weren't important, or at least they were unrelated to health. New research shows conclusively that nutrient deficiencies and dependencies do exist when people try to maintain their health on three meals a day using the "four food groups."

You just cannot get all the vitamins and minerals you need from the standard three meals a day.

When your body has been assaulted by stress, drugs, pollutants, injury, or sickness, you lose nutrients more quickly than usual. If these are not replaced, your ability to withstand stressors or fight off disease is reduced.

With all of our machines and gadgets, most of us do far less manual labor than we did at any other time in the history of humankind. With so many labor-saving devices, we need fewer calories. That means we reduce our food intake.

That's not to say we lose weight. In fact, most of us probably gain weight because we cannot get the nutrition that we need through our food alone.

It is nearly impossible to get all the nutrients we need without taking supplements.

Pollutants in the air, food and water put a stress on all of us. As a result, we require more vitamins and minerals to support the enzyme systems that aid in discharging these toxins.

Those sweet, salty, crunchy "empty calorie" foods we eat rob the body of the nutrients we need for digestion and absorption. In addition, food sensitivities and yeast infections damage intestinal lining cells so that even when we do eat nutrient-dense food, the absorption from these foods is limited.

So supplements are important even for those of us who do eat the right amounts of the best foods. You and everyone you know needs ALL of the 90 essentials nutrients every day and in a form that is absorbable. Give your body the raw materials that it needs, and it will do amazing things.

Educate yourself, and learn the truth about nutrition, and the odds are that you're going to save yourself an enormous amount of unnecessary misery. You're going to save yourself a gob of money. And you're going to have many, many, many healthful years of life.

It will definitely help you to educate yourself about nutrition instead of relying on your doctors.

Don't let somebody else, even a doctor—no, especially a doctor—determine your future.

You can make those determinations yourself, and you can do a far better job than anybody else can. After all, this is your life to live. Live it wisely, and live it well.

For more information about nutrition, please visit our website, www.truthaboutnutrition.com, or call 1-800-592-2933.

Made in the USA
Columbia, SC
17 February 2021